Recent Advances in Hallux Rigidus Surgery

Guest Editor

MOLLY SCHNIRRING-JUDGE, DPM, FACFAS

CLINICS IN PODIATRIC MEDICINE AND SURGERY

www.podiatric.theclinics.com

Consulting Editor
THOMAS ZGONIS, DPM, FACFAS

April 2011 • Volume 28 • Number 2

SAUNDERS an imprint of ELSEVIER, Inc.

W.B. SAUNDERS COMPANY
A Division of Elsevier Inc.

1600 John F. Kennedy Boulevard • Suite 1800 • Philadelphia, Pennsylvania 19103-2899

http://www.theclinics.com

CLINICS IN PODIATRIC MEDICINE AND SURGERY Volume 28, Number 2
April 2011 ISSN 0891-8422, ISBN-13: 978-1-4557-0495-8

Editor: Patrick Manley

Clinics in Podiatric Medicine and Surgery (ISSN 0891-8422) is published quarterly by Elsevier Inc., 360 Park Avenue South, New York, NY 10010-1710. Months of issue are January, April, July, and October. Business and Editorial Offices: 1600 John F. Kennedy Blvd., Ste. 1800, Philadelphia, PA 19103-2899. Customer Service Office: 3251 Riverport Lane, Maryland Heights, MO 63043. Periodicals postage paid at NewYork, NY and additional mailing offices. Subscription prices are $270.00 per year for US individuals, $385.00 per year for US institutions, $137.00 per year for US students and residents, $324.00 per year for Canadian individuals, $477.00 for Canadian institutions, $384.00 for international individuals, $477.00 per year for international institutions and $193.00 per year for Canadian and foreign students/residents. To receive student/resident rate, orders must be accompanied by name of affiliated institution, date of term, and the *signature* of program/residency coordinator on institution letterhead. Orders will be billed at individual rate until proof of status is received. Foreign air speed delivery is included in all *Clinics* subscription prices. All prices are subject to change without notice. POSTMASTER: Send address changes to *Clinics in Podiatric Medicine and Surgery*, Elsevier Health Sciences Division, Subscription Customer Service, 3251 Riverport Lane, Maryland Heights, MO 63043. **Customer Service: 1-800-654-2452 (US). From outside of the US, call 314-447-8871. Fax: 314-447-8029. E-mail: JournalsCustomerService-usa@elsevier.com (for print support); JournalsOnlineSupport-usa@elsevier.com (for online support).**

Reprints. For copies of 100 or more of articles in this publication, please contact the Commercial Reprints Department, Elsevier Inc., 360 Park Avenue South, New York, NY 10010-1710. Tel.: 212-633-3812; Fax: 212-462-1935; E-mail: reprints@elsevier.com.

Clinics in Podiatric Medicine and Surgery is covered in *MEDLINE/PubMed (Index Medicus)* and *EMBASE/Excerpta Medica.*

Printed and bound by CPI Group (UK) Ltd, Croydon, CR0 4YY

Transferred to Digital Print 2011

CLINICS IN PODIATRIC MEDICINE AND SURGERY

CONSULTING EDITOR
THOMAS ZGONIS, DPM, FACFAS

Contributors

CONSULTING EDITOR

THOMAS ZGONIS, DPM, FACFAS
Director, Podiatric Surgical Residency and Reconstructive Fellowship Programs;
Chief, Division of Podiatric Medicine and Surgery; Associate Professor, Department
of Orthopedic Surgery, The University of Texas Health Science Center at San Antonio,
San Antonio, Texas

GUEST EDITOR

MOLLY SCHNIRRING-JUDGE, DPM, FACFAS
Director, Research and Publications, Cleveland Clinic Foundation–Kaiser Permanente
Foundation Podiatric Residency Program, Cleveland, Ohio; Adjunct Faculty, Colleges
of Podiatric Medicine and Ohio University, Athens; Faculty, Graduate Medical Education,
Mercy Health Partners, Toledo, Ohio; Private Practice, North West Ohio Foot and Ankle
Institute, LLC, Serving Ohio and Michigan, Lambertville, Michigan

AUTHORS

MARTHA A. ANDERSON, DPM
Private Practice, Department of Surgery, Grady Memorial Hospital, Delaware, Ohio

ALLAN BOIKE, DPM, FACFAS
Section Head, Podiatric Medicine and Surgery, Director of Podiatric Medical and Surgery
Residency Training, Foot and Ankle Center, Orthopaedic and Rheumatologic Institute,
Cleveland Clinic, Cleveland, Ohio

GEORGEANNE BOTEK, DPM, FACFAS
Medical Director, Diabetic Foot Center; Staff, Department of Orthopaedic Surgery,
Orthopaedic and Rheumatologic Institute, Cleveland Clinic, Cleveland, Ohio

BRADLY W. BUSSEWITZ, DPM, AACFAS
Fellow, Orthopedic Foot and Ankle Center, Westerville, Ohio

WILLIAM T. DECARBO, DPM, AACFAS
Attending Physician, Orthopedic Foot and Ankle Center, OhioHealth, Westerville, Ohio;
The Orthopedic Group, Belle Vernon, Pennsylvania

BRIAN L. FREEMAN, DPM
Resident, Foot and Ankle Residency Program, Cleveland Clinic Foundation–Kaiser
Permanente; Department of Orthopedics/Podiatry, Cleveland Clinic Foundation,
Cleveland, Ohio

MELISSA M. GALLI, DPM, MHA
Podiatric Surgical Resident, Department of Orthopaedics, The Ohio State University
Medical Center, Columbus, Ohio

MARK A. HARDY, DPM, FACFAS
Director, Foot and Ankle Residency Program, Cleveland Clinic Foundation–Kaiser Permanente; Director, Foot and Ankle Trauma Service, Kaiser Permanente – Ohio Region, Cleveland; Department of Podiatric Surgery, Kaiser Permanente Foundation, Cleveland Heights, Ohio

DAVE HEHEMANN, DPM, PGY-2
Cleveland Clinic Foundation–Kaiser Permanente, Cleveland, Ohio

GINA A. HILD, DPM
Resident DPM, Podiatry Section, Department of Orthopaedic Surgery, Cleveland Clinic Hospital, Cleveland Clinic Foundation–Kaiser Permanente Medical Center, Cleveland, Ohio

CHRISTOPHER F. HYER, DPM, FACFAS
Fellowship, Co-Director; Advanced Foot and Ankle Reconstructive Surgical Fellowship, Orthopedic Foot and Ankle Center, Westerville, Ohio

TIM LEVAR, DPM
Resident, Podiatric Surgery, Cleveland Clinic Foundation, Cleveland, Ohio

JEFFREY LUPICA, DPM
Resident, Department of Podiatric Medicine and Surgery, Kaiser Permanente/Cleveland Clinic Foundation, Kaiser Permanente/Cleveland Clinic, Mentor, Ohio

MICHAEL C. MCGLAMRY, DPM
Attending DeKalb Medical Center; Faculty, Podiatry Institute, Decatur, Georgia

PATRICK J. MCKEE, DPM
Staff, Department of Orthopaedic Surgery, Cleveland Clinic Foundation, Cleveland Clinic, Cleveland, Ohio

SEAN MCMILLIN, DPM
Resident, Cleveland Clinic/Kaiser Permanente, Department of Orthopaedics Podiatric Residency Training Program, Cleveland, Ohio

JARED L. MOON, DPM
Second Year Resident, DeKalb Medical Center, Decatur, Georgia

CRYSTAL L. RAMANUJAM, DPM
Clinical Instructor and Postgraduate Research Fellow, Division of Podiatric Medicine and Surgery, Department of Orthopaedic Surgery, University of Texas Health Science Center at San Antonio, San Antonio, Texas

MOLLY SCHNIRRING-JUDGE, DPM, FACFAS
Director, Research and Publications, Cleveland Clinic Foundation–Kaiser Permanente Foundation Podiatric Residency Program, Cleveland, Ohio; Adjunct Faculty, Colleges of Podiatric Medicine and Ohio University, Athens; Faculty, Graduate Medical Education, Mercy Health Partners, Toledo, Ohio; Private Practice, North West Ohio Foot and Ankle Institute, LLC, Serving Ohio and Michigan, Lambertville, Michigan

THOMAS ZGONIS, DPM, FACFAS
Director, Podiatric Surgical Residency and Reconstructive Fellowship Programs; Chief, Division of Podiatric Medicine and Surgery; Associate Professor, Department of Orthopedic Surgery, The University of Texas Health Science Center at San Antonio, San Antonio, Texas

Contents

an emphasis on the procedure to prepare a successful arthrodesis, and expounds on technical nuances including those associated with fixation devices.

THE CLINICS ARE NOW AVAILABLE ONLINE!

Access your subscription at:
www.theclinics.com

Foreword

Hallux Rigidus

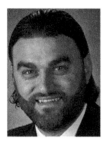

Thomas Zgonis, DPM
Consulting Editor

When degenerative changes occur to the first metatarsal phalangeal joint (MTPJ), regardless of etiology, we broadly classify the condition as *Hallux Rigidus*. Despite this simple term, the etiology of the condition varies greatly based on the lower extremity biomechanics and has truly been controversial and debated throughout the literature for at least two decades. This debate does not exist over secondary arthritic changes as a result of previous trauma, inflammatory arthritic conditions, and/or iatrogenic insult. Even though the proposed biomechanical causes of hallux rigidus are debatable, a long first metatarsal and metatarsal primus elevatus are the underlying basis for the majority of the osteotomies that were initially designed to treat this condition. The structural abnormalities and/or altered biomechanics that lead to primary osteoarthritis of the first MTPJ are what fuels this continued debate and the paradoxes of procedure selection. Despite the true etiology, when symptomatic arthritis does occur, the resultant functional disability and the effect on a patient's quality of life are significant.

Logically, a joint-sparing procedure for hallux rigidus would be preferred. Cheilectomy is currently the most commonly utilized procedure with or without osteotomy of the proximal phalanx for the treatment of mild and moderate osteoarthritis of the first MTPJ. When cheilectomy fails or when severe osteoarthritis of the first MTPJ is present, the gold standard is a first MTPJ arthrodesis. This is not to discredit the advances in surgical selection for joint-sparing procedures such as joint replacement, interpositional arthroplasty, arthrodiastasis, and biologic joint resurfacing. Performing a fusion of the first MTPJ is by no means a simple surgery. The procedure carries a risk of painful malunion and nonunion that concerns every foot and ankle surgeon that performs this procedure on a regular basis.

The invited authors have done a spectacular job in creating this edition that not only reviews the current literature but also thoroughly discusses emerging technology and

Clin Podiatr Med Surg 28 (2011) xi–xii
doi:10.1016/j.cpm.2011.03.007

insight to guide procedure selection along with technical tips and pearls for both conservative and surgical management of this debilitating condition. I thank you for your continuous efforts and your outstanding submissions.

Thomas Zgonis, DPM
Division of Podiatric Medicine and Surgery
Department of Orthopaedic Surgery
The University of Texas Health Science Center
at San Antonio
7703 Floyd Curl Drive–MSC 7776
San Antonio, TX 78229, USA

E-mail address:
zgonis@uthscsa.edu

Preface

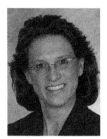

Molly Schnirring-Judge, DPM
Guest Editor

The on-going contemplation of degenerative joint disease deformity about the first metatarsal phalangeal joint (MTPJ) and its treatment has given rise to much research and advancement in modern technology over time. While osteochondral disease and injury can potentially affect any joint, there is a frequency of occurrence of hallux limitus and hallux rigidus among athletes and otherwise active patients that cannot be ignored.

The spectrum of disease in the progression from hallux limitus to hallux rigidus has proven to be an enigma of sorts among foot pathologies. While it may seem intuitive that the correlation between clinical and radiographic findings should direct procedure selection, we have learned that these parameters often fall short of the actual severity of the osteochondral injury found intraoperatively. When the true extent of the intra-articular injury is realized (often much more severe than radiographs predict), problem-solving is immediately shifted back to the common sense perspective: what are the patient's goals and expectations in function and how can I best achieve these given the nature and extent of this irreversible joint disease?

For this edition of *Clinics in Podiatric Medicine and Surgery (CPMS)*, I have been given the unique opportunity to work with the residency program directors and surgeons of the Cleveland Clinic Foundation–Kaiser Permanente Podiatric Residency Program in Cleveland, Ohio as well as the The Orthopedic Foot and Ankle Center in Westerville, Ohio. In this edition of *CPMS*, the contributing authors have prepared information and shared thought processes that naturally evolve when considering the spectrum of pathology from hallux limitus to hallux rigidus. Their unique insights lend themselves to a well-rounded and inspired approach to understanding this insidiously progressive degenerative joint disease of the first MTPJ. The collective experience of these surgeons provides an interesting and up-to-date interpretation of the disease process and the treatment modalities available to address the spectrum of degenerative change and dysfunction associated with it. A review of the biomechanics and etiology of hallux limitus provides an interesting prelude to the pathology of the sesamoid apparatus and how that contributes to the process of joint dysfunction. Considering current concepts in surgery for dysfunction about the first MTPJ includes the most recent trends and technology in both hallux abducto valgus and hallux rigidus surgery. The wide range of surgical options for these conditions includes the latest

Clin Podiatr Med Surg 28 (2011) xiii–xiv
doi:10.1016/j.cpm.2011.04.001
0891-8422/11/$ – see front matter © 2011 Elsevier Inc. All rights reserved.

approaches and most modern instrumentation as the topics evolve from updated techniques in HAV surgery through multiplanar osteotomies, resurfacing techniques, arthrodiastasis, the modified cheilectomy, implants. Ultimately the first MTPJ arthrodesis is described as a practical procedure with predictable outcomes for end stage disease and chronic pain. It is my hope that this edition will serve as a useful desk reference for practical applications in the treatment of dysfunction about the first MTPJ.

Respectfully submitted to the readership,

Molly Schnirring-Judge, DPM
North West Ohio Foot and Ankle Institute, LLC
7581 Secor Road
Lambertville, MI 48144, USA

E-mail address:
mjudegmolly@aim.com

Etiology, Pathophysiology, and Staging of Hallux Rigidus

Georgeanne Botek, DPM[a,b],*, Martha A. Anderson, DPM[c]

KEYWORDS

• Hallux rigidus • Hallux limitus • Classification • Osteoarthritis
• First metatarsophalangeal joint

A normal first metatarsophalangeal joint (MTPJ) range of motion is assessed during the propulsive phase of gait and should approximate 65° to 75° of dorsiflexion. Given our aging population, the foot and ankle surgeon should expect to encounter cases of osteoarthritis of the first MTPJ on an increasing basis. Understanding this condition, which causes less than the normal range of sagittal plane motion in the first MTPJ, is critical, given that it currently affects 1 in 45 middle-aged persons[1] and 35% to 60%[2] of the population older than 65 years. Even though this pathologic condition is commonly treated by the foot and ankle surgeon, the cause of first MTPJ osteoarthritis or hallux limitus is not completely understood. Numerous causative factors have been suggested, yet few well-designed studies have thoroughly investigated risk factors for hallux limitus and demonstrated the progression from hallux limitus to advanced degenerative changes found in hallux rigidus in which a stiff ankylosed joint results. The current literature fails to tie anatomic abnormalities to the long-term success of a single surgical procedure. The foot and ankle surgeon determines that a specific cause exists and selects a surgical procedure based on this premise, but little evidence truly exists that one procedure is better than another. More importantly, regardless of the procedure performed, there is no long-term clinical evidence reported in the literature that suggests the cause of this disease has truly been arrested. The historical literature suggests that the cause may range from external factors, such as improper or constrictive shoe gear, to inherited genetic traits and

The authors have nothing to disclose.

[a] Department of Orthopaedic Surgery, Diabetic Foot Clinic, Cleveland Clinic, 9500 Euclid Avenue A-40, Cleveland, OH 44195, USA
[b] Diabetic Foot Clinic, Cleveland Clinic, 9500 Euclid Avenue A-40, Cleveland, OH 44195, USA
[c] Private Practice, Department of Surgery, Grady Memorial Hospital, 29 Grandview Avenue, Delaware, OH 43015, USA
* Corresponding author. Department A-40, 9500 Euclid Avenue, Cleveland, OH 44195.
E-mail address: botekg@ccf.org

Clin Podiatr Med Surg 28 (2011) 229–243
doi:10.1016/j.cpm.2011.02.004
0891-8422/11/$ – see front matter © 2011 Elsevier Inc. All rights reserved.

congenital defects. The current literature emphasizes radiographic anatomy and patterns of subchondral bone destruction often relating them to the mechanics of the first ray, midfoot, rearfoot, and ankle complexes. Much of history has been refuted more recently, and much current thought is challenged by others seeking the same truths. Examining the cause of hallux limitus allows the foot and ankle surgeon to understand the best surgical and nonsurgical options. By fully understanding the nature and mechanism of the condition, physicians more likely are able to demonstrate superior functional outcomes based on a truthful understanding.

HISTORY OF HALLUX LIMITUS

More than a century has passed since degenerative arthritis of the first MTPJ was initially described by Davies-Colley[3] and given the name hallux limitus by Cotterill.[4] Another descriptive term is hallux rigidus, the condition resulting in functional limitation of motion of the hallux.[5] The term dorsal bunion[6,7] describes the development of a large dorsal osteophyte, whereas hallux flexus[3] and hallux equinus[8,9] similarly describe the great toe being placed in a position of flexion. As the great toe becomes increasingly plantar, the metatarsal appears elevated, which is aptly referred to as metatarsus primus elevatus.[10–12]

Early descriptions of hallux limitus often focused on the presence of osteochondritis dissecans in adolescents.[3,13–16] In 1888, Davies-Colley[3] attributed the onset to pressure of a short rigid boot on a long great toe. In 1936, McMurray[13] similarly identified ill-fitting shoes as the cause of this adolescent pathology when he wrote, "In adolescence the condition is usually found in association with a long foot which is narrower than normal, and examination of the great toe shows that the power of dorsiflexion is lost."

CAUSES OF HALLUX LIMITUS
Excessive Length

Evaluating the length pattern of the first metatarsal as a causative factor in the etiology of hallux limitus is all across the board when one turns to the investigators in the literature on this topic. A long first metatarsal is considered a primary contributing factor in the development of hallux limitus.[17] Root and colleagues[18] listed 5 main causes of hallux limitus, the first being excessive length of the first metatarsal. Nilsonne[17] postulated that a long first metatarsal restricts plantar flexion and increases compression of the first MTPJ. Varied and often contradictory findings are reported in more recent literature. After reviewing 180 radiographs of hallux rigidus, Beeson and colleagues[19] demonstrated that the first metatarsal was appreciably (ie, more than 1 mm) longer than the second metatarsal in only 37% of instances, whereas the first metatarsal was longer than the third metatarsal 73% of the time. In another radiographic analysis, Munuera and colleagues[20] concluded that although there was a trend in increased anatomic length of the first metatarsal in hallux limitus, it was not statistically significant. Bryant and colleagues[21] did not find any significant difference between groups, and Zgonis and colleagues[22] reported that the first metatarsal was significantly shorter in those with hallux limitus than that in controls. Simply put, stating that the first metatarsal length is a causative factor in the development of hallux limitus is at best a nebulous finding. Perhaps one might even deduce that the first metatarsal length pattern has nothing to do with the etiology of hallux limitus.

Hypermobility and Metatarsus Primus Elevatus

Root and colleagues[18] cited hypermobility as a second cause of hallux limitus. As a consequence of increased subtalar joint pronation, the lateral column of the foot becomes unstable in midstance and the propulsive stages of gait, thus depriving the peroneus longus of its plantar flexion on the first ray. A functional limitation of hallux dorsiflexion may follow with a first metatarsal that dorsiflexes and inverts, rather than having the mechanical advantage of plantar flexion.

The role of the sagittal plane alignment of the first metatarsal in the development of hallux limitus is somewhat complex.[23] The concept of metatarsus primus elevatus was first described by Lambrinudi[14] in 1938 based on a single patient, "Mrs M." This surgeon observed an unsteady gait and an elevated medial column and surgically addressed the problem with bone grafting and plantar flexion of the first ray. Because of this successful case study, elevatus was cited as a cause of hallux limitus. But one may question whether the elevatus was the result of a painful arthritic great toe causing an antalgic or compensatory gait or was it simply because of instability. Similarly, Jack[24] also describe metatarsus primus elevatus but again with less than abundant objectivity or proof.

Root, too, cited metatarsus primus elevatus as a third cause of hallux limitus.[18] Since then, several other investigators have also suggested that metatarsus primus elevatus may be a causative factor.[23] Horton and colleagues[5] reported a larger difference in the first and second metatarsal declination angles in individuals with hallux limitus compared with controls, indicating a dorsiflexed metatarsal relative to the second. Similarly, Bryant and colleagues[21] reported that the lateral intermetatarsal angle was increased in the group with hallux limitus.

However, not all recent investigators agree with the idea of metatarsus elevatus as a common cause in the development of hallux limitus. Meyer and colleagues[25] examined metatarsus primus elevatus in a group of 120 randomly selected foot radiographs. The diagnosis of hallux rigidus was made radiographically in 22 cases on the basis of the presence of dorsal osteophytes, joint space narrowing, and flattening of articular cartilage. No direct relationship existed between the amount of elevation and the severity of hallux limitus. Another large radiographic study points out that the mean values for elevation of the first ray in patients with mild or moderate hallux rigidus were nearly identical to those in the control group. An average of 8 mm of metatarsus primus elevatus is a normal finding in patients with hallux rigidus as well as in normal subjects. Horton and colleagues[5] reviewed lateral weight-bearing radiographs from 81 patients with hallux rigidus and a control population. The results revealed that the mean values for elevation of the first ray in patients with hallux limitus were nearly identical to those in the control group. More support for this finding was found in a cross-sectional study that examined 180 feet radiologically to find that 89% of metatarsals did not demonstrate elevation greater than the 8 mm reported as normal.[19]

More broadly evaluating first ray elevatus, Camasta[9] viewed metatarsus primus elevatus and hallux equinus as being codependent on either uncompensated varus or pes planovalgus versus the earlier analyses that looked at metatarsus primus elevatus as an isolated condition. Camasta describes an elevated medial column with a hallux assuming a resting position of equinus to provide medial weight-bearing stability in an uncompensated varus. Similarly, with a pes planovalgus foot type, the flexors of the hallux forcefully contract in an attempt to provide medial column stability to resist unstable rearfoot.

Other Causes

Immobility of the first ray is a fourth causative factor in hallux limitus as described by Root and colleagues and Chang and Camasta.[18,26] Medial column degenerative joint disease at the metatarsocuneiform joint may be an end-stage complication of chronic subtalar joint pronation, a congenital problem, or a condition associated with a previous deformity, such as hallux valgus, trauma, a systemic arthritis (such as rheumatoid, gout, or psoriatic), or a septic arthritis of the medial column.[26] This condition is termed secondary arthritis because hallux limitus is associated with degenerative change due to various other metabolic diseases. Primary osteoarthritis, meaning localized arthritic process of the first MTPJ, has been recognized as causing hallux limitus.[26,27] Arthritis can propagate with disruption to the first MTPJ anatomy after hallux valgus surgery or can result in a dorsally displaced metatarsal after a base wedge osteotomy. Root and colleagues[18] recognize osteoarthritis and trauma as other causative factors for hallux limitus.

Histologic Changes

Even when trauma is not mentioned as the cause or when the condition is bilateral, which occurs 64% of the time,[19] similar anatomic changes are evident. Histologic evidence indicates a traumatic etiology, and a mechanism of injury is suggested. McMaster[7] cites common microscopic appearances regardless of reported histories of injury: a cleavage lesion in the articular cartilage without any attached subchondral bone located in the central dome of the metatarsal head. Histologic preparations of the lesion in the metatarsal head are almost entirely cartilaginous, and the changes in the subchondral bone suggest that they are secondary to increased stress or trauma. Trauma, whether acute or chronic, has always been emphasized as a cause of hallux limitus yet is associated in merely 22% of cases.[19] If the great toe is stubbed, the forced extension and axial compression of the dorsal lip on the proximal phalanx impinges the convex head of the first metatarsal between the apex of the dome and the dorsal margin.[7] Such a tangential force applied acutely or repetitively in minor incidences can produce an osteochondral fracture or a cartilaginous cleavage in the metatarsal head.[7] The natural course of this disorder is typical of other degenerative osteoarthritic processes with progression of the osseous articular changes leading to limitation of motion and disruption of normal first MTPJ function.[10] Characteristic chondral and osteochondral lesions occur at the central first metatarsal head dome, and the subsequent classic horseshoe-shaped dorsal collar of bone that is present accounts for the limitation of dorsiflexion but relatively unrestricted plantar flexion (**Fig. 1**).[7] Although progression from hallux limitus to hallux rigidus commonly increases stiffness and decreases range of motion at the MTPJ, one study surveying 24 feet points out that most individuals in this study did not have progression of pain or symptoms over a 12-year period.[28] This study analyzed the radiographic outcomes along with patient satisfaction of nonoperative care of hallux limitus. Most patients with hallux limitus rated their pain as staying the same over a 12-year period, despite significant deterioration of joint space noted radiographically. So, despite the natural history of hallux rigidus with radiographic worsening, pain did not correlate with the majority in this group whose average age began at 53 years. Ninety-two percent claimed that their pain had not substantially changed since the time of original diagnosis.[28] Although there are limitations to radiographic analysis, it is hard to deny the valor of subjective satisfaction if it has been accurately reported. (Radiographic pictures are limited in their ability to comprehensively evaluate hallux limitus. A 2-dimensional view has its limitations.)

RADIOGRAPHIC PARAMETERS IN HALLUX LIMITUS

The most common objective evaluation of hallux limitus has been first MTPJ radiological assessment (anteroposterior, lateral, oblique, and forefoot axial or sesamoid views) because the determinants of normal and abnormal conditions have been well

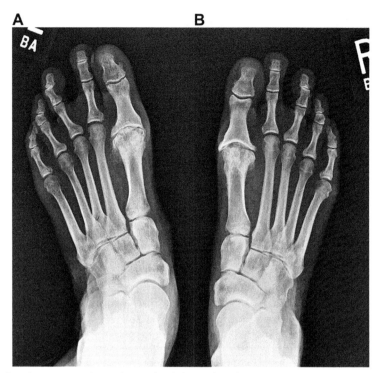

Fig. 1. (*A, B*) Intraoperative radiograph of classic dorsal wear pattern in hallux limitus with a horseshoe collar of dorsal osteophytoses and base of proximal phalanx.

defined. Radiographically, the diagnosis is characterized by dorsal exostoses of the first metatarsal head and base of the proximal phalanx, flattening of the metatarsal head, joint space narrowing, and osteophytic lipping of the MTPJ (**Fig. 2**).[29] The etiology of hallux limitus may be varied, and although numerous investigators have corroborated anatomic abnormalities associated with this condition, only few agree on findings that may be risk factors for developing hallux limitus. A square rather than round metatarsal head may predispose toward joint compression during propulsion and lead to degenerative joint disease.[30–32] Increased width of the first metatarsal and proximal phalanx as a morphologic feature noted on plain radiographs suggest that this could predispose individuals to having a square articular surface (**Fig. 3**).[20] One study evaluating radiological parameters correlated increased hallux interphalangeal angle with increased first MTPJ narrowing (**Fig. 4**).[19] Munuera and colleagues[20]

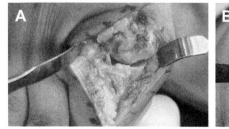
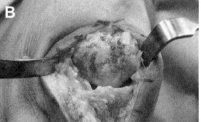

Fig. 2. (*A, B*) Weight-bearing lateral radiographs of hallux limitus.

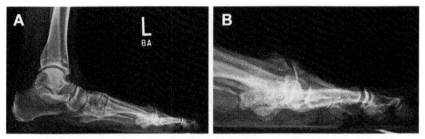

Fig. 3. (*A, B*) Bilateral anteroposterior radiographs demonstrating widening of the proximal phalanx, narrowing of the joint space and medial, and lateral joint impingement.

concluded that a longer metatarsodigital segment was seen more frequently in hallux limitus radiographs.[33] Yet another study found a single significant radiological finding in hallux limitus: increased medial angulation of the second MTPJ with increased hallux rigidus grade (**Fig. 5**).[34] Sesamoid pathology has been radiologically documented in 65% of cases of hallux limitus.[19] Sesamoid hypertrophy and proximal displacement have been hypothesized, but Munuera and colleagues[20] did not find proximal migration when looking at 183 samples of weight-bearing dorsal plantar radiographs, 115 normal feet, and 68 feet with hallux limitus. This radiographic analysis found longer sesamoids in individuals with hallux limitus than in controls, but it may be significant to note that the subjects' ages ranged from 20 to 29 years in this study Again, elevation of the first metatarsal and an elongated first metatarsal are not overwhelmingly supported in numerous radiographic analyses,[5,19,21,22] and the

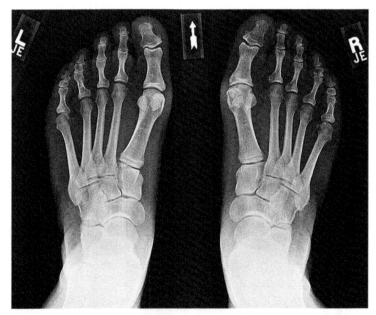

Fig. 4. Bilateral anteroposterior radiographic view with right first MTPJ changes more consistent with hallux limitus. Yet, note bilateral increase in hallux interphalangeal angle, wide metatarsal, and proximal phalanx. A flattened squaring-off of the metatarsal head is noted.

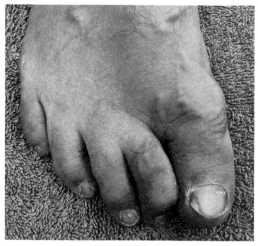

Fig. 5. Appearance of second MTPJ adduction in association with the dorsal spurring of the first MTPJ.

causative factors that lead to the development of most adult-onset first MTPJ arthrosis are unknown[5,11] or, perhaps, multifactorial. To deduce meaning from the investigators cited on this topic, the foot and ankle surgeon must individually assess the radiographs of this growing patient population and take into consideration that there may not be a single overwhelming cause or a dominant procedure that effectively addresses hallux limitus. Historical views have been challenged. Investigators, of late, seem to want to disprove existing dogma rather than discount met primus elevatus as a biomechanical etiology, combine clinical perception with radiographic assessment, and discern etiologies along with procedural choices.

KINEMATIC PATHOPHYSIOLOGY

Certain pathomechanics can be expected as a result of or as a cause of hallux limitus. Whether one believes in metatarsus primus elevatus as a probable causative factor, unanimous agreement for a dorsal prominence of the distal first metatarsal must be appreciated, particularly in end-stage hallux rigidus. Intraoperative findings reveal a periarticular osseous ridge of hypertrophied bone extending medially, dorsally, and laterally in a U-shaped collar of bone along the articular cartilage (see **Fig. 1**). Many patients have concomitant osteophyte formation on the medial, dorsal, and lateral surfaces of the base of the proximal phalanx (see **Fig. 3**). These 2 osseous prominences mechanically block motion and lead to jamming of the joint during the arc of motion.[35] Some patients present to the office because of an acute exacerbation of chronic pain in the MTPJ. This pain may be caused by a fracture of a portion of the metatarsal or phalangeal osteophyte that leads to a loose fragment of bone within the joint. In general, pain, stiffness, and swelling are the classic presentation, with some patients also complaining of occasional paresthesias.

Kinematic analyses of the first MTPJ in hallux limitus reveal a decrease in the arc of motion, with relatively normal plantar flexion but reduced dorsiflexion (**Fig. 6**).[10,35] The normal physiologic dorsiflexion of the first MTPJ implemented in gait is estimated to be 65° to 75°. Without such motion, secondary pathologic foot problems might be hypothesized.[29,36–38] Kinematic studies of hallux limitus demonstrate increased

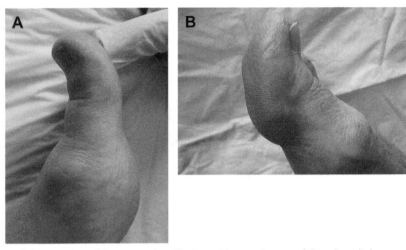

Fig. 6. (*A*) Limitation of first MTPJ dorsiflexion with prominence of dorsal medial metatarsal exostoses. (*B*) Remarkable plantar hallux interphalangeal joint prominence/bursitis noted in this case of hallux limitus.

plantar foot pressures to the hallux as well as laterally, although increased plantar first MTPJ pressures in symptomatic first MTPJ osteoarthritis has also been documented (**Fig. 7**).[15] With the great toe being in a flexed or equinus position, pressure in stance and propulsion transfers laterally and distally. Bryant and colleagues[21] found that those with hallux limitus displayed significantly higher mean pressures under the hallux, lesser toes, and the third and fourth metatarsal heads. Comparing individuals with radiographically confirmed osteoarthritis of the first MTPJ with controls, greater maximum force and peak pressures under the hallux and under the lesser toes were demonstrated, concluding that in hallux limitus, an oblique axis is used in

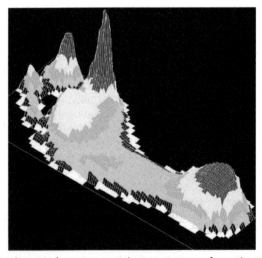

Fig. 7. Examined by dynamic foot pressure/plantar pressure of a patient with hallux limitus demonstrating elevated plantar pressures of the hallux interphalangeal joint and first MTPJ.

push-off, which subjects the lateral forefoot and toes to increased loading and results in hyperextension of the interphalangeal joint of the hallux.[29]

CLASSIFICATION AND STAGING

Hallux limitus and rigidus can be classified based on clinical assessment, radiographic findings, or a combination of both. Multiple systems have been developed for this purpose, and surgical recommendations are formulated based on the severity or classification of the deformity. The current literature fails to report surgical outcomes based on preoperative radiographic parameters.

Clinically, hallux rigidus can be divided into functional and structural categories. Nilsonne and Cohn and Kanat[17,39] described primary and secondary hallux rigidus. The investigators correlated primary hallux rigidus with metatarsus primus elevatus and found that this was typically seen in younger male patients. Secondary hallux rigidus was attributed to posttraumatic changes or degenerative arthritis in elderly patients.

Functional hallux rigidus can be differentiated from structural hallux rigidus by clinical examination. Normally, 65° to 75° of dorsiflexion occurs during propulsion at the first MTPJ.[18] Patients with a functional or primary rigidus have a normal amount of dorsiflexion in the non–weight-bearing condition.[40–42] However, when the foot is loaded, a decreased range of motion at the first MTPJ is apparent. Patients with a structural or secondary hallux rigidus have limited range of motion in both the loaded and unloaded positions.[40]

Several classifications for structural hallux rigidus exist, as many as 18 different classification systems have been identified.[43] One of the most widely recognized classification systems was developed by Regnauld.[44] This system takes both clinical and radiographic findings into consideration (**Table 1**). Some of the variation in this classification from one reference to the next may be attributable to the fact that the classification itself was translated from a foreign language (French) to English.[43]

Hattrup and Johnson[45] also developed a classification system based on radiographic findings. Grades I to III were assigned based on the severity of osteophyte formation around the first MTPJ and associated joint space narrowing (**Table 2**). All of the patients underwent cheilectomy in this study, and the failure rate was 15% for grade I, 31.8% for grade II, and 37.5% for grade III.[45]

Kellgren and Lawrence[46] coauthored an atlas of osteoarthritis for grading the severity of joint disease. This atlas was initially meant for generalized degenerative joint disease, but various investigators have adapted this classification to the foot

Table 1 Regnauld classification	
Grade I	Mild limitation of dorsiflexion, mild dorsal spurring, pain, no sesamoid involvement, subchondral sclerosis, mild sesamoid enlargement
Grade II	Broadening and flattening of the metatarsal head and base of the proximal phalanx, focal joint space narrowing, structural first ray elevatus, osteochondral defect, sesamoid hypertrophy
Grade III	Worsening loss of joint space, near ankylosis, extensive osteophyte formation, osteochondral defects, extensive sesamoid hypertrophy, with or without joint mice

Data from Regnauld B. Disorders of the great toe. In: Elson R, editor. The foot: pathology, aetiology, seminology, clinical investigation and treatment. New York: Springer-Verlag; 1986. p. 269–81.

Table 2	
Hattrup and Johnson classification	
Grade I	Mild to moderate osteophyte formation, preserved joint space
Grade II	Moderate osteophyte formation, joint space narrowing, subchondral sclerosis
Grade III	Marked osteophyte formation, loss of visible joint space, with or without subchondral cyst formation

Data from Hattrup SJ, Johnson KA. Subjective results of hallux rigidus following treatment with cheilectomy. Clin Orthop Relat Res 1988;226:182–91.

specifically (**Table 3**).[47] This system is similar to the one developed by Hattrup and Johnson but includes a grade 0 for patients without clinical or radiographic evidence of disease.

Another more recent atlas has been developed specifically for the joints in the foot. Menz and colleagues[48] analyzed 5 different foot joints, including the first MTPJ. Each joint was assessed radiographically on 2 views and given a value from 0 to 3 based on the severity of osteophyte formation and joint space narrowing (**Table 4**). No clinical correlation was performed in the development of this atlas.

Roukis and colleagues[34] implemented a novel radiographic classification as well (**Table 5**). These investigators describe 4 categories with progressive worsening severity and even noted sesamoid osteopenia in some patients with grade III arthritic changes (see **Fig. 3**). This is one of the few prospective studies in which surgery was undertaken and the intraoperative findings were correlated with the preoperative grade of deformity. In this study, it was found that grade I findings (metatarsus primus elevatus, subchondral sclerosis, and hallux equinus) correlated with articular erosion less than 50% intraoperatively, whereas grade III findings (dorsal exostosis, lateral joint flare, joint space narrowing, sesamoid hypertrophy, and subchondral cyst formation) corresponded to articular cartilage loss greater than 50% on the metatarsal head. There were no significant findings between radiographic evaluation and intraoperative findings in patients classified with grade II disease.[34]

Hanft and colleagues[49] used a classification system based on objective radiographic findings.[9,40] The investigators developed subgroups of the later stages if osteochondral defects, loose bodies, or subchondral cyst formation was present (**Table 6**). This system uniquely attempted to correlate surgical procedure choice based on the radiographic findings and stage of severity of hallux rigidus. For patients with grade I hallux rigidus, procedure recommendations were cheilectomy, metatarsal

Table 3	
Kellgren and Lawrence classification	
Grade 0	No degenerative changes
Grade 1	Questionable osteophytes, no joint space narrowing
Grade 2	Osteophytes with possible joint space narrowing
Grade 3	Joint space narrowing, moderate osteophyte formation, mild subchondral sclerosis
Grade 4	Severe joint space narrowing, subchondral cysts, severe osteophyte formation, moderate to severe subchondral sclerosis

Data from Kellgren JH, Lawrence JS. Atlas of standard radiographs: the epidemiology of chronic rheumatism, vol. 2. Oxford (United Kingdom): Blackwell Scientific; 1963.

Table 4
The Menz and colleagues classification

Value	Osteophyte Formation	Joint Space Narrowing
0	Absent	None
1	Small	Definite
2	Moderate	Severe
3	Severe	Joint fusion at any part of the joint

Data from Menz HB, Munteanu SE, Landorf KB, et al. Brief report. Radiographic classification of osteoarthritis in commonly affected joints of the foot. Osteoarthritis Cartilage 2007;15:1333–8.

Table 5
The Roukis and colleagues classification

Grade I	Metatarsus primus elevatus with hallux equinus, periarticular subchondral sclerosis, minimal dorsal exostosis, minimal flattening of the metatarsal head
Grade II	Moderate dorsal exostosis and flattening of the metatarsal head, minimal joint space narrowing, lateral metatarsal head erosion with or without exostosis, sesamoid hypertrophy, with or without subchondral cysts or loose bodies
Grade III	Severe dorsal exostosis, focal joint space narrowing, subchondral cyst formation, loose bodies, traction enthesopathic sesamoid hypertrophy with immobilization-induced osteopenia
Grade IV	Excessive exostosis with trumpeting of the metatarsal head, proximal phalanx base, and sesamoid apparatus; minimal or absent joint space; sesamoid ankylosis; hallux interphalangeal and/or first metatarsal medial cuneiform arthrosis

Data from Roukis TS, Jacobs PM, Dawson DM, et al. A prospective comparison of clinical, radiographic, and intraoperative features of hallux rigidus. J Foot Ankle Surg 2002;41:76–95.

Table 6
The Hanft and colleagues classification

Grade I	Metatarsus primus elevatus, mild spurring with dorsal hypertrophy of the metatarsal head and proximal phalangeal base, subchondral sclerosis
Grade II	Grade I plus broadening and flattening of the first metatarsal head and base of the proximal phalanx, decreased joint space, sesamoid hypertrophy, lateral osteophyte formation on the first metatarsal head
Grade IIB	Grade II plus osteochondral defects, subchondral cyst formation, subchondral fracture, or loose bodies
Grade III	Grade II plus severe flattening of the metatarsal head and proximal phalanx, severely decreased joint space, dorsal and lateral osteophyte formation, extensive sesamoid hypertrophy
Grade IIIB	Grade III plus osteochondral defects, loose bodies, or subchondral cyst formation

Data from Hanft JR, Mason ET, Landsman AS, et al. A new radiographic classification for hallux limitus. J Foot Ankle Surg 1993;32:397–404.

or phalangeal osteotomy, and sesamoid release. Those with grade II hallux rigidus had the same recommendation plus optional joint decompression (ie, Regnauld procedure). Grade IIB added chondroplasty and loose body removal as an option. Grade III added total joint arthroplasty, and Grade IIIB added arthrodesis or Keller osteotomy.[49]

Coughlin and Shurnas[50] have a unique classification system in that range of motion, radiographic findings, and clinical symptoms are all included.[51] This classification was meant to ease nonsurgical and surgical treatment options and provide optimum outcomes after surgery (**Table 7**). Beeson and colleagues[43] found that when comparing classification systems for hallux rigidus, no gold standard exists to which

Table 7
The Coughlin and Shurnas classification

	Range of Motion	Radiographic Findings	Clinical Findings
Grade 0	DF 40°–60° and/or 10%–20% loss compared with normal side	Normal or minimal	No pain, stiffness, loss of passive motion on examination
Grade 1	DF 30°–40° and/or 20%–50% loss compared with normal side	Dorsal spurring, minimal joint narrowing, minimal sclerosis, and metatarsal flattening	Mild or occasional pain and stiffness, pain at extreme DF and/or PF on examination
Grade 2	DF 10°–30° and/or 50%–75% loss compared with normal side	Dorsal, lateral, and possible medial osteophytes; flattened metatarsal head; no more than one-fourth dorsal joint space involvement on lateral view; mild to moderate joint space narrowing and sclerosis; sesamoids typically not involved	Moderate to severe pain and stiffness, pain before maximal DF and/or PF on examination
Grade 3	DF ≤10° and/or 75%–100% loss compared with normal side, loss of PF	As in grade 2, but substantial narrowing, possible cystic changes, more than one-fourth dorsal joint space involvement, sesamoid hypertrophy or cystic changes	Near-constant pain and stiffness, pain throughout range of motion on examination
Grade 4	Grade 3 plus pain at mid–range of motion on examination		

Abbreviations: DF, dorsiflexion; PF, plantar flexion.
Data from Coughlin MJ, Shurnas PS. Hallux rigidus: grading and long-term results of operative treatment. J Bone Joint Surg Am 2003;85:2072–88; and Shurnas PS. Hallux rigidus: etiology, biomechanics, and nonoperative treatment. Foot Ankle Clin 2009;14:1–8.

new systems can be compared. However, the investigators did find that the system used by Coughlin and Shurnas most closely approximated such a standard. The only drawback of this system was that it was applied retrospectively in the investigators' study.

Many similarities exist between these classification systems, but noted differences abound. Because no true gold standard for the classification of hallux rigidus exists currently, future investigators will have the responsibility to either validate a current classification or develop and implement a new validated and reliable classification that can be easily applied both in practice and for research purposes. Why a single classification system is not widely recognized remains unclear. Hallux limitus is a common diagnosis with well-defined radiographic and clinical findings and is the second most common disorder that affects the first MTPJ after hallux abductovalgus.[39] We as a profession should strive to implement a standardized and validated classification system that aids in both nonoperative treatment and procedure selection for surgical correction.

SUMMARY

Hallux limitus is a common degenerative disease affecting the first MTPJ. It is seen increasingly with age with most recent reports showing a mean age of onset of 44 years and with women affected slightly more commonly than men.[2,10,19,23,31]

Pain, swelling, and stiffness are most often the presenting symptoms. Surgical as well as nonsurgical treatments have been effective at eliminating symptoms. To achieve better treatment outcomes, understanding the pathophysiology, assessing patient risk factors, and identifying etiologic agents better equip the foot and ankle surgeon in managing this condition.

REFERENCES

1. Gould N, Schneider W, Ashikago T. Epidemiological survey of foot problems in the continental United States: 1978–1979. Foot Ankle 1980;1:8–10.
2. Van Saase JL, Van Romunde LK, Cats A, et al. Epidemiology of osteoarthritis: Zoetermeer survey. Comparison of radiological osteoarthritis in a Dutch population with that in 10 other populations. Ann Rheum Dis 1989;48:271–80.
3. Davies-Colley N. On contraction of the metatarsophalangeal joint of the great toe (hallux flexus). Trans Clin Soc Lond 1887;20:165–71.
4. Cotterill JM. Stiffness of the great toe in adolescents. Br Med J 1887;1(1378): 1158.
5. Horton GA, Park YW, Myerson MS. Role of metatarsus primus elevatus in the pathogenesis of hallux rigidus. Foot Ankle Int 1999;20:777–80.
6. Lapidus PW. "Dorsal bunion": its mechanics and operative correction. J Bone Joint Surg 1940;22:627–37.
7. McMaster MJ. The pathogenesis of hallux rigidus. J Bone Joint Surg Br 1978;60: 82–7.
8. Rzonca E, Levitz S, Boue B. Hallux equinus. J Am Podiatry Assoc 1984;74:390–3.
9. Camasta CA. Hallux limitus and hallux rigidus: clinical examination, radiographic findings, and natural history. Clin Podiatr Med Surg 1996;13:423–48.
10. Shereff MJ, Baumhauer JF. Current concepts review. Hallux rigidus and osteoarthrosis of the first metatarsophalangeal joint. J Bone Joint Surg Am 1998;80: 898–908.
11. Mann RA. Hallux rigidus. Instr Course Lect 1990;39:15–21.

12. Myerson MS, Horton GA, Park YW. The role of metatarsus elevatus in the pathogenesis of hallux rigidus. Read at the Specialty Day Meeting of the American Orthopaedic Foot and Ankle Society. Atlanta, February 25, 1996.
13. McMurray TP. Treatment of hallux valgus and rigidus. Br Med J 1936;3943:218–21.
14. Lambrinudi C. Metatarsus Primus Elevatus. Proceedings of the Royal Society of Medicine, Section of Orthopaedics, volume XXXI, 1273, Sectional page 51, January 4, 1938.
15. Duckworth SD. Reports of societies. Br Med J 1887;728.
16. Goodfellow J. Aetiology of hallux rigidus. Section of Orthopaedics. Proc R Soc Med 1966;59:821–4.
17. Nilsonne H. Hallux rigidus and its treatment. Acta Orthop Scand 1930;1:295–303.
18. Root ML, Orien WP, Weed JH. Motion at specific joints of the foot. In: Root SA, editor. Normal and abnormal function of the foot. 1st edition. Los Angeles (CA): Clinical Biomechanics Corporation; 1977. p. 46–60, 350–70.
19. Beeson P, Phillips C, Coor S, et al. Cross-sectional study to evaluate radiological parameters in hallux rigidus. Foot (Edinb) 2009;19:7–21.
20. Munuera PV, Dominguez G, Castillo JM. Radiographic study of the size of the first metatarsophalangeal segment in feet with incipient hallux limitus. J Am Podiatr Med Assoc 2007;97:46–8.
21. Bryant A, Tinley P, Singer K. A comparison of radiographic measurements in normal, hallux valgus, and hallux limitus feet. J Foot Ankle Surg 2000;39:39–43.
22. Zgonis T, Jolly GP, Garbalosa JC, et al. The value of radiographic parameters in the surgical treatment of hallux rigidus. J Foot Ankle Surg 2005;44:184–9.
23. Zammit GV, Hylton BM, Muneaunu SE. Structural factors associated with hallux limitus/rigidus: a systematic review of case control studies. J Orthop Sports Phys Ther 2009;39:733–42.
24. Jack EA. The aetiology of hallux rigidus. Br J Surg 1940;27:492–7.
25. Meyer JO, Nishon LR, Weiss L, et al. Metatarsus primus elevatus and the etiology of hallux rigidus. J Foot Surg 1987;26:237–41.
26. Chang TJ, Camasta CA. Hallux limitus and hallux rigidus. In: Banks AS, McGlamry ED, editors. McGlamry's comprehensive textbook of foot and ankle surgery. 3rd edition. Philadelphia: Lippincott Williams & Wilkins; 2001. p. 679–711.
27. Kashuk KB. Hallux rigidus, hallux limitus, and other functionally limiting disorders of the great toe joint: background and treatment and case studies. J Foot Surg 1975;14:45.
28. Smith RW, Katchis SD, Ayson LC. Outcomes in hallux rigidus patients treated nonoperatively: a long-term follow-up study. Foot Ankle Int 2000;21:906–14.
29. Zammit GV, Menz HB, Munteanu SE, et al. Plantar pressure distribution in older people with osteoarthritis of the first metatarsophalangeal joint (hallux limitus/rigidus). J Orthop Res 2008;26:1665–9.
30. Brahm SM. Shape of the first metatarsal head in hallux rigidus and hallux valgus. J Am Podiatr Med Assoc 1988;78:300–4.
31. Coughlin MJ, Shurnas PS. Hallux rigidus: demographics, etiology, and radiographic assessment. Foot Ankle Int 2003;24:731–43.
32. DuVries H. Static deformities. In: DuVries H, editor. Surgery of the foot. St Louis (MO): C.V. Mosby; 1959.
33. Munuera PV, Dominguez G, Lafuente G. Length of the sesamoids and their distance from the metatarsophalangeal joint space in feet with incipient hallux limitus. J Am Podiatr Med Assoc 2008;98:123–9.
34. Roukis TS, Jacobs PM, Dawson DM, et al. A prospective comparison of clinical, radiographic, and intraoperative features of hallux rigidus. J Foot Ankle Surg 2002;41:76–95.

35. Shereff MJ, Bejjani FJ, Kummer FJ. Kinematics of the first metatarsophalangeal joint. J Bone Joint Surg Am 1986;68:392–8.
36. Joseph J. Range of motion of the great toe in men. J Bone Joint Surg Br 1954;36: 450–7.
37. Buell T, Green DR, Risser J. Measurement of the first metatarsophalangeal joint range of motion. J Am Podiatr Med Assoc 1988;78:439–48.
38. Mann RA, Hagy JL. The function of the toes in walking, jogging, and running. Clin Orthop Relat Res 1979;142:24–9.
39. Cohn I, Kanat IO. Functional limitation of motion of the first metatarsophalangeal joint. J Foot Surg 1984;23:477–84.
40. Lichniak JE. Hallux limitus in the athlete. Clin Podiatr Med Surg 1997;14:407–26.
41. Scherer PR, Sanders J, Eldredge DE, et al. Effect of functional foot orthoses on first metatarsophalangeal joint dorsiflexion in stance and gait. J Am Podiatr Med Assoc 2006;96:474–81.
42. Hall C, Nester CJ. Sagittal plane compensations for artificially induced limitation of the first metatarsophalangeal joint. J Am Podiatr Med Assoc 2004;94:269–74.
43. Beeson P, Phillips C, Corr S, et al. Classification systems for hallux rigidus: a review of the literature. Foot Ankle Int 2008;29:407–14.
44. Regnauld B. Disorders of the great toe. In: Elson R, editor. The foot: pathology, aetiology, seminology, clinical investigation and treatment. New York: Springer-Verlag; 1986. p. 269–81.
45. Hattrup SJ, Johnson KA. Subjective results of hallux rigidus following treatment with cheilectomy. Clin Orthop Relat Res 1988;226:182–91.
46. Kellgren JH, Lawrence JS. Atlas of standard radiographs: the epidemiology of chronic rheumatism, vol. 2. Oxford (United Kingdom): Blackwell scientific; 1963.
47. Mahiquez MY, Wilder FV, Stephens HM. Positive hindfoot valgus and osteoarthritis of the first metatarsophalangeal joint. Foot Ankle Int 2006;27:1055–9.
48. Menz HB, Munteanu SE, Landorf KB, et al. Brief report. Radiographic classification of osteoarthritis in commonly affected joints of the foot. Osteoarthritis Cartilage 2007;15:1333–8.
49. Hanft JR, Mason ET, Landsman AS, et al. A new radiographic classification for hallux limitus. J Foot Ankle Surg 1993;32:397–404.
50. Coughlin MJ, Shurnas PS. Hallux rigidus: grading and long-term results of operative treatment. J Bone Joint Surg Am 2003;85:2072–88.
51. Shurnas PS. Hallux rigidus: etiology, biomechanics, and nonoperative treatment. Foot Ankle Clin 2009;14:1–8.

Evaluation and Biomechanics of the First Ray in the Patient with Limited Motion

Gina A. Hild, DPM[a],*, Patrick J. McKee, DPM[b]

KEYWORDS

• Biomechanics • First ray • Hallux limitus

Biomechanics, in particular biomechanics of the first ray, has evolved in the years since pioneers such as Morton and Root first described their theories. Evidence-based medicine is now finding flaws with previously believed concepts that were developed by these pioneers. Dudley Morton was a surgical anatomist who graduated from Hahemann Medical College in 1907 and served as faculty at Yale. He is credited with his theory of disordered foot function, which is based on the premise that a short first ray (or metatarsus atavicus), associated with hypermobility of the first ray, was a common cause of foot dysfunction. This foot type is now known as the Morton foot type. Morton considered that a short first metatarsal would prevent the first ray from contacting the ground during gait and that this function would be taken over by the longer second metatarsal and cause a lateral shifting of weight. In the past 80 years, many investigators[1–4] have refuted the initial conclusions proposed by Dr Morton. It is now generally accepted that a short metatarsal does not, by itself, lead to foot disorder or dysfunction. Hypermobility is also now known to be much less common than originally believed and has also been proved to be present in the healthy human foot in addition to the foot with pathologic process. Increased lateral foot pressures in the Morton foot type have since been confirmed in the literature.[5]

Merton Root, DPM, is credited with starting the Department of Orthopedics at the California College of Chiropody, which later became the California College of Podiatric Medicine. He is commonly associated with many important discoveries regarding foot function, such as the introduction of the concept of neutral subtalar joint position,

The authors have nothing to disclose.
Links for permission: none.
[a] Department of Orthopaedic Surgery, Cleveland Clinic Foundation/Kaiser Permanente Residency Program, 9500 Euclid Avenue, Desk A40, Cleveland, OH 44195, USA
[b] Department of Orthopaedic Surgery, Cleveland Clinic Foundation, Cleveland Clinic, 9500 Euclid Avenue, Desk A40, Cleveland, OH 44195, USA
* Corresponding author.
E-mail address: hildg@ccf.org

Clin Podiatr Med Surg 28 (2011) 245–267
doi:10.1016/j.cpm.2011.03.003
0891-8422/11/$ – see front matter © 2011 Elsevier Inc. All rights reserved.

although others refute this claim.[6] He is also credited with developing the ideas of neutral casting techniques that included instruction on the development and manufacturing of orthotic devices. Root also developed a list of 8 biophysical normals, which predicted physiologic normal foot function and structure. This list progressed into a classification scheme for foot and ankle deformities. Lee[7] presented a 138-page full review of Root function and podiatric biomechanics. Root's ideas have since been challenged in the literature and it is now believed that such normal feet may not truly exist.[6,8]

McPoil and Hunt[8] proposed that 3 main concerns exist with Root theory. First, they identify that the measurement techniques used by Root were unreliable. Second, they identify that inconclusive evidence has been presented to support Root's criteria for normal foot alignment. A third concern was expressed regarding the position of the subtalar joint between midstance and heel-off during walking. The investigators proposed a more reliable tissue stress model as an alternative to Root theory. This model is discussed later.[8]

ANATOMIC BIOMECHANICS OF THE FIRST RAY

The first metatarsophalangeal joint (MTPJ) comprises 4 articulating surfaces including the first metatarsal, the proximal phalanx, and fibular and tibial sesamoid bones, which are all contained within a synovial capsule. The joint is a ginglymoarthrodial type with the ginglymus or hinge motion occurring during the first 20 to 30 degrees of dorsiflexion and the arthrodial or gliding motion occurring during the remainder of propulsion. This joint has been described as a hammock within which the first metatarsal head sits and rolls.[9] It is also described by Hetherington and colleagues[10] as a dynamic acetabulum. The first metatarsal and medial cuneiform make up the osseous components of the first ray.[2,11,12] Others describe it as comprising the anatomic articulations between the first metatarsal, medial, and intermediate cuneiforms and navicular bones.[13]

Many muscles are involved in first ray function and motion. The extensor hallucis longus (EHL) originates from the interosseous membrane and anterior surface of the tibia and inserts into the distal phalanx. Its main contribution to first ray function is to promote extension stability of the first MTPJ and interphalangeal joint (IPJ) of the hallux. Another function is to exert a posterior force from the distal phalanx to its more proximal structures, converting it into a rigid beam during propulsion before toe-off. It also assists during swing phase to promote hallux dorsiflexion, clearing the toe from ground surfaces. An extra slip of the EHL tendon also exists, called the extensor hallucis capsularis. This small slip is believed to take the tension out of the first MTPJ during dorsiflexion. This small structure is present in approximately 88% of the population and can be used in tendon augmentation and grafting.[14] The extensor hallucis brevis originates in the sinus tarsi and inserts into the proximal dorsal aspect of the proximal phalanx. It is the most medial slip of the extensor digitorum brevis muscle. Its functions include stabilizing the hallux posteriorly against the first metatarsal and the first metatarsal posteriorly against the lesser tarsus. This muscle functions primarily during midstance and early propulsion. The abductor hallucis provides abductory stability to the hallux. It also provides posterior stabilization of the hallux toward the first metatarsal. Propulsive stability of the hallux against the ground and plantarflexion of the first ray and stabilization of the first metatarsal head against the ground are other functions performed by this muscle.[11]

The adductor hallucis muscle comprises both an oblique head and a transverse head. These 2 muscles are described in the literature as having distinct functions. An oblique head originates at the bases of metatarsals 2, 3, and 4 and inserts into the inferior surface of the proximal phalanx after converging with the transverse head and encapsulating the fibular sesamoid.[15] The main functions of this tendon are to stabilize the hallux in adduction and to exert posterior force of the proximal phalanx against the first metatarsal head. Another function includes stabilizing the proximal phalangeal base against the ground during propulsion. A transverse head, the transverse pedis muscle, also exists, which originates from the lateral plantar aspect of the base of the proximal phalanx and inserts along the course of the deep transverse intermetatarsal ligament (DTIL). It provides transverse stability of the transverse arch of the foot primarily through stabilization of plantar MTPJs during propulsion and prevents elongation of the DTIL.[11]

The flexor hallucis longus tendon originates on the posterior surface of the fibula and interosseous membrane and inserts into the plantar surface of the base of the distal phalanx of the hallux. Its contributions to first ray function include plantarflexing the hallux against the ground and converting the hallux to a rigid beam during propulsion. In addition, it provides stabilization of the distal phalanx posteriorly against proximal phalanx of hallux. The flexor hallucis brevis (FHB) originates on the plantar surface of the cuboid and lateral, or third, cuneiform and inserts into the plantar base of the proximal phalanx with 2 heads each of which encapsulate the tibial and fibular sesamoids. This muscle serves to stabilize the base of the proximal phalanx of the hallux against the ground during propulsion and also provides posterior stabilization of the hallux against first metatarsal head during propulsion. Another function of the FHB is to stabilize first, second, and third metatarsals against their corresponding cuneiforms.[11]

The peroneus longus tendon passes obliquely under the foot and functions to stabilize the foot in a plantar and lateral position. There are 4 main functions of the peroneus longus tendon during closed kinetic chain. Its main function is to stabilize the first ray in a posterior and lateral direction toward the lesser tarsus and the first metatarsal head against the ground. Stabilization occurs toward the end of midstance and into propulsion. The second function includes the shifting of weight from the lateral foot to the medial foot during early propulsion. Other functions include limiting ankle joint dorsiflexion, aiding in heel lift, and assisting ankle joint plantarflexion during the propulsive phase.[9]

Peroneus longus function during closed kinetic chain was studied in cadaver models by Johnson and Christensen.[16] Progressive loads were applied to the tibia and fibula of these specimens and tarsal motion was measured. They found significant frontal plane motion in the direction of eversion with higher and higher loading of the proximal segments. Less significant angular changes were also noticed within the sagittal and transverse planes of the medial column. Findings were that the peroneal longus tendon exhibits a locking effect on the first ray of the foot against the rest of the foot.[16] The cadaver study was then repeated in patients who had undergone Lapidus fusion of the first metatarsocuneiform and increased dorsiflexion of the talus and frontal plane eversion were noted in the corrected cadaver specimens, indicating a more stable first ray. They believed this was also secondary to the effects of the peroneal longus tendon and its effect of stabilizing the medial column.[16]

Continued study was performed by Johnson and Christensen[17] to determine the effects that the Achilles tendon/equinus would have on first ray function. Cadaver studies were performed with increasing levels of Achilles tendon tensile loads to simulate equinus. It was determined that, as heel tightness increased, more flattening of the medial arch was observed, although results were not significant. They did find a significant relationship with an inverted first metatarsal and equinus of the Achilles tendon.

The main conclusion of the study was that equinus resulted in destabilization of peroneus longus muscle function.[17]

The tibialis anterior muscle originates on the lateral aspect of the tibial shaft and interosseous membranes and inserts into the plantar surface of the medial cuneiform and base of first metatarsal. The main functions of this muscle include inverting the foot and dorsiflexing the ankle.[11]

Ligamentous support structures of the first ray include the tibial collateral, tibial sesamoid, and plantar tibial sesamoidal ligaments medially and the fibular collateral, fibular sesamoidal, and plantar fibular sesamoidal ligaments laterally.[15] Electromyographic studies have not found a significant contribution of intrinsic or extrinsic muscular activity during stance phase, attributing most first ray stability during stance secondary to ligamentous support.[18] First ray stability is mainly a function of the plantar fascia and the first metatarsocuneiform ligament (MCL).[19,20] Mizel[20] studied the strength of the plantar first MCL by isolating and severing it in 5 cadaver specimens. All specimens were noted to have at least a 5-mm dorsal displacement with instability following loss of this important ligament. They concluded that this structure was essential in the support of the first metatarsal during weight bearing, and that any injury could result in lateral shifting of weight and increased stress under the lesser metatarsals.

AXIS OF MOTION OF THE FIRST RAY

In 1954, Hicks[2] was one of the first to describe a single axis of first ray motion that was suspended through the mid-dorsum of the foot over the base of the third metatarsal to the tuberosity of the navicular. He determined a 22-degree range of motion (ROM) and found that with flexion of the first ray pronation would occur and that with extension of the first ray supination would occur.[2] Ebisui[21] also performed studies on the first ray axis that verified Hicks' prior study.

This same axis of motion was described by Root as passing from the proximal medial dorsal aspect of the talonavicular joint to the distal lateral plantar aspect of the third metatarsal cuneiform joint. This first ray axis is almost parallel to the transverse plane limiting motion in this direction and angles about 45 degrees from both the sagittal and frontal planes, allowing for most motion to occur within these planes. Archlike rotary movement occurs around this axis and results in inversion when dorsiflexed and eversion while plantarflexed, which was similar to Hicks' earlier findings.[11]

A high-gear and low-gear axis were described through the works of Bojsen-Moller[1] after studying the skeletons of 25 human feet and comparing them with gorilla, chimpanzees, and orangutans. The first metatarsal was described as being part of the high-gear, transverse axis that included the second metatarsal. The collaboration of these metatarsals made up the foundation of faster or higher speeds in pedal gait among humans. The remaining oblique axis was composed of metatarsals 2 to 5 and slower pedal gait would progress over this axis.[1]

NORMAL AND ABNORMAL FIRST RAY MOTION AND FUNCTION

For walking to occur, several detailed collaborative pedal events must occur. Normal gait stance phase is initiated by heel-off. Once the heel lifts off the ground, the subtalar joint supinates and the peroneus longus fires, stabilizing the medial column next to the remainder of the lateral foot. As the peroneus longus fires, the first metatarsal head plantarflexes and the sesamoid apparatus becomes a pulley. Weight now transfers laterally in the forefoot from the second and subsequent lesser metatarsals. As the weight transfers, the proximal phalanx is allowed to dorsiflex in the sagittal plane, allowing propulsion to occur around it. The hallux should not move once it purchases the ground and acts as a lever over which the remainder of the foot can pass. Adequate hallux dorsiflexion on the first metatarsal is essential for normal function and gait. It is the purchase of the toe against the ground that creates the shear force necessary for propulsion to occur.[22]

Roukis and colleagues[13] performed a 1996 study in which they evaluated first ray dorsiflexion and its effects on overall first ray mobility. Three positions of the first ray were studied in normal test subjects. They found a trend toward decreased ability of the hallux to dorsiflex with subsequent elevation of the first ray. Dorsiflexion decreased by 19% when the first ray was elevated by only 4 mm and then decreased by 36% when the first ray was elevated by 8 mm. The conclusions of the study were based on the premise that when the first ray dorsiflexes it also inverts. An increase in the amount of dorsiflexion available also results in an increase in inversion. It is the inversion that is responsible for increasing transverse plane motion and this, theoretically, leads to hallux abductus as opposed to hallux rigidus disorders.[13] A similar study was performed on cadaver limbs by Perez and colleagues,[23] which determined that sagittal plane motion would be decreased when the first ray was in a position of eversion. Sagittal plane motion also decreased when the first ray was in a position of inversion, but this was not found to be significant.[23]

How much motion is necessary at the first MTPJ for normal function to occur is the subject of considerable debate. Hiss,[24] in 1937, was one of the first to relate that the average first MTPJ ROM was 90 degrees, with dorsiflexion and plantarflexion being divided equally at 45 degrees each. Joseph,[25] in 1954, described the normal motion to be an average of 90.8 degrees in open kinetic chain. The average normal of 90 degrees still holds true today. Kelikian[26] then determined that the average ROM was 70 degrees, but did not mention whether this value was open or closed kinetic chain. In 1977, Root and colleagues[11] described approximately 65 degrees of dorsiflexion as necessary for proper first ray function. Mann and Hagy,[27] in 1979, determined that 30 to 40 degrees of dorsiflexion were necessary to clear the toes from dragging on the ground during closed kinetic chain. They also suggested that 70 to 90 degrees of dorsiflexion would be obtained at the first MTPJ in a normally functioning foot. In the same year, Bojsen-Moller[28] found that 20 to 30 degrees of dorsiflexion were noted at heel strike and an average of 58 degrees of dorsiflexion when walking at 100 steps per minute.

Shereff and colleagues[29] studied the kinematics of the first ray with 15 fresh-frozen cadaver limbs disarticulated below the knee. Six subjects were identified as having normal anatomy, 6 had hallux valgus deformities, and 3 had hallux rigidus. They noted a normal ROM to be, on average, 111 degrees in the sagittal plane, with 76 degrees being dorsiflexion and 34 degrees being plantarflexion. They found limitation in dorsiflexion among cadavers with hallux rigidus. Diseased cadavers were found to have eccentrically located instant centers of rotation. They also found increased motion of the medial sesamoid bone compared with that of the lateral sesamoid. Within this study they also confirmed the hypothesis that a normal amount of transverse plane motion occurs at the first MTPJ during propulsion. They found this motion in a normal individual to be approximately 2 mm. In the hallux rigidus population, this was found to be about 1 mm. They considered this to be the end result of contracted collateral ligaments and joint capsule.[29] Similar ranges of motion were found by Buell[30] in 1988 in a comparison of clinical and radiographic evaluations. Normal dorsiflexion was 90 degrees when unassisted clinically and 89 degrees radiographically. In all instances, angulation was obtained from the first metatarsal shaft, to which reproducible measurement were attributed.

In 1989, Hetherington and colleagues[10] stated that 60 to 70 degrees of first MTPJ motion during propulsion were essential for normal gait to occur. He also described

4 instant centers of rotation about the first metatarsal head that occurred about an arc that was present in areas of increased stress. This finding contradicted prior interpretations that motion of the first MTPJ was that of a simple hinged joint. Motion occurring within the joint was described in this study as rolling when metatarsal dorsiflexion begins, followed by sliding during metatarsal plantarflexion and then compression near the end of propulsion. They described the joint as that of a dynamic acetabulum[10] and concurred with Kelikian's[26] prior description that referred to the joint as a hammock. Hetherington and colleagues[31] completed another study, in 1990, with normal subjects during toe-off and found an average functional dorsiflexion of the first MTPJ to be 50.56 degrees. Hopson and colleagues[32] also studied 4 clinical tests to determine optimal first MTPJ ROM and also found that 65 degrees was required for normal walking to occur.

Perez and colleagues[23] proposed that the first ray exhibited a locking mechanism akin to those in the talonavicular and calcaneocuboid joints. They postulated that an increase in frontal plane motion would secondarily affect sagittal plane motion of the first MTPJ. First ray motion was evaluated in cadaver limbs and was found to be lower when everted (7 mm) versus the ROM when inverted (18 mm). The investigators considered that this suggested the presence of a locking position within the first ray.[23]

Plantar pressures have been measured recently in elderly patients with radiographically confirmed osteoarthritis and decreased clinical ROM within the first MTPJ. As expected, peak pressures were significantly higher (23% higher) compared with those without hallux limitus/rigidus. They also found an average increase in maximum forces of 34% under the hallux in this population. No other areas of the foot were found to have significant change in load bearing as a result. The conclusions were that the higher pressures result in plantar callus formation and hyperextension of the hallux interphalangeal joint (HIPJ).[33]

SHAPE OF THE FIRST METATARSAL HEAD

Numerous studies have been performed to determine whether the shape of the metatarsal head predisposes an individual to the development of hallux limitus, rigidus, or hallux valgus.[9,34–38] Schweitzer and colleagues[38] found a positive correlation between a flat metatarsal head in 16.7% and a long metatarsal in 9% in his study of magnetic resonance imaging findings among patients with hallux rigidus. Coughlin and Shurnas[39] also found that 93/127 (73%) of his patients with hallux rigidus possessed a flat or chevron-shaped metatarsal head.

Multiple investigators have also determined that a round metatarsal head predisposes an individual to hallux abducto valgus (HAV).[34–37,40] It is also suggested that a square or ridge-shaped metatarsal head predisposed an individual to the development of hallux limitus or rigidus.[9] Okuda and colleagues[37] studied 60 patients with HAV to determine the recurrence rate of bunion surgery on those with varying metatarsal head shapes. They found that a round articular and lateral surface of the metatarsal head was more consistent with developing bunions, as well as increasing the risk of recurrence of bunion after surgical intervention.[37]

Mancuso and colleagues[36] discussed a zero-plus first metatarsal and its relationship to bunion development. A zero-plus metatarsal is at least the same length or longer than the second metatarsal and was found to be clinically significant in the development of HAV. They also found a significant relationship between the round metatarsal and hallux valgus population, finding 91% of their HAV patients with a round metatarsal head.[36]

THE WINDLASS MECHANISM

Hicks[41] was one of the first to describe first ray motion through the effects of a windlass mechanism. He compared the foot with a winding cable (the plantar fascia) wrapped around the drum of a windlass (metatarsophalangeal joint) that is pulled by a lever (the hallux). Dorsiflexion of the toe results in pulling and shortening of the plantar fascia, compressing the medial column and resulting in a lateral shift of weight toward the outside of the foot.[41]

Kappel-Bargas and colleagues[42] studied the in vivo role of the windlass mechanism during gait. They discovered that windlass was active during first MTPJ extension. Activation of the windlass mechanism was delayed in those with greater overall rear foot eversion. This delay was believed to be the result of poor midfoot stabilization in the pronated population. Aquino and Payne[43] disputed this finding in their 2001 study, in which they found disruption of the windlass mechanism in individuals exhibiting inverted forefoot-to-rearfoot relationships (pronated forefoot), medial deviation of subtalar joint axis, and lower navicular drift. They did not find a positive correlation between pronated foot type and alteration in windlass effects. However, lack of objective data and subjective observational results establish a need for using caution when interpreting these results.[43]

Functional stability of the medial column was assessed through the works of Rush and colleagues[44] in 2000. They performed a cadaver study that assessed corrected and uncorrected transverse plane deformities of the first metatarsal. They discovered that, when the first metatarsal was in a corrected position, the windlass mechanism was engaged with a 26% increase in plantarflexion. They summarized that this mechanism was more functional when the sesamoid apparatus, metatarsal, and hallux were adequately aligned. They also suggested that procedures such as Keller, sesamoid removal, or overaggressive shortening of distal osteotomy would result in a damping effect that would function to destabilize the first ray. This destabilization would result secondary to plantar fascial and peroneus longus dysfunction as they lose the ability to stabilize the first ray.

Mechanical engineering models have also been developed to analyze the windlass mechanism. Kinetics is the study of force that causes movement. It is more descriptive when discussing how an anatomic structure can move, accounting for outside stresses within the environment. Fuller[45] applied this model to the plantar fascia in order to explain disorders of the foot. Newtonian physics models were applied to the foot and mathematical comparisons of an arch with a tension band attached to a drum with a lever were made.[45]

Ultrasound examinations of diabetic patients with and without neuropathy were performed in a study by D'Ambrogi and colleasgues[46] in 2005. Plantar aponeurosis was noted to be thickened in diabetic patients with and without neuropathy. The thickening was postulated to be secondary to an increase in protein glycosylation of the plantar fascia that is seen in other collagen-rich tissues of the body. Rigidity of the plantar fascia leads to excessive contracture through the windlass mechanism, resulting in increased pressure under the forefoot.[46]

MEDIAL COLUMN, METATARSUS PRIMUS ELEVATUS, AND HYPERMOBILITY: THE DEBATE

The medial column is supported through the interaction of the first metatarsocuneiform (MTC), the naviculocuneiform (NC), and talonavicular (TN) joints. Medial column evaluation of these joints was performed through the works of Roling and colleagues.[47] They discovered that the NC joint contributed the most motion to the first ray, resulting in 50% of its motion. The first MTC also contributed significantly with 41%, and the talonavicular contributed only 9% of first ray motion. Further evaluation of arthrodesis of these joints, including arthrodesis of the first metatarsocuneiform-intercuneiform determined that, regardless of the fusion being performed, all significantly decreased first ray motion. All of the joints within the medial column were intimately related and fusion of any of them locked up the medial column. Faber and colleagues[48] repeated the cadaver test of Roling and colleagues[47] in individuals with HAV deformity and found the main contributing joint to motion was the first met-cuneiform joint, with 57% of the motion.

Lapidus arthrodesis was also studied by Avino and colleagues,[49] who found significant changes in both talo–first metatarsal angles and medial cuneiform height after surgery. Phillips and colleagues[50] determined that the NC joint was responsible for most sagittal plane plantarflexory motion of the first ray during propulsion.

Associations between metatarsus elevatus and hallux limitus have been described in the literature,[51–53] but others refute this claim.[39,54,55] Camasta[52] describes a situation in which proximal uncompensated varus deformity of the foot exists. In order for the foot to meet the ground, the hallux plantarflexes, producing a hallux equinus. This hallux equinus leads to dorsal impingement. They also discuss flexible flatfoot as contributing to medial column instability, which results in a similar splinting of the hallux causing articular cartilage destruction and arthritis.[52] Banks and colleagues[51] suggest that flexible pes planovalgus results in a degree of hypermobility within the medial column of the foot. The plane of motion in which the compensation occurs determines whether a hallux abductovalgus or hallux limitus/rigidus results. They describe transverse or frontal plane compensation as leading to HAV deformity and sagittal plane compensation leading to hallux limitus/rigidus.[51] Meyer and Bryant and colleagues[54,55] did not find significant associations between the first metatarsal elevation in those with hallux limitus, disputing results of prior studies.

Metatarsus elevatus, and its association with hallux limitus and rigidus, was studied by Coughlin and Shurnas[39] in 2003. They described a physiologic normal value on lateral radiograph to be equal to or less than 8 mm. They did not determine that metatarsus elevatus was seen in their preoperative population of 110 individuals. An average metatarsal elevation of 5.5 mm was found within their preoperative study participants. However, they did find that this elevation would routinely decrease after cheilectomy, especially among those with less severe disease (stage I or II). Advanced degeneration of articular cartilage was associated with residual elevatus in a few of their patients. They also considered that, if the joint had progressed to the point at which elevation of the first ray was noted before surgery, this would be an indication for arthrodesis, which always decreased elevatus after surgery.[39] Meyer[55] refuted the claim that elevatus was associated with disorders in his study in which a normal population had up to 7-mm elevatus without pathologic effect.

Hypermobility of the first ray has often been defined in the literature as an increase in sagittal plane motion of more than 4 mm.[56] It is now believed that hypermobility should also be identified in the transverse plane[48] and that an increase in transverse plane motion of more than 8 mm within a joint should be considered hypermobile.[56] This feature is often seen in individuals with Ehlers-Danlos and Marfan syndromes.[12,56] Hypermobility is more commonly associated in the literature with hallux valgus deformity compared with hallux limitus/rigidus.[12,56] Rush and colleagues[44] describe hypermobility as a continuum that results when the windlass mechanism is not engaged secondary to a poorly aligned first ray. The misalignment of the first ray results in an inability of the anterior tibial tendon to create tension around the medial column and, as a result, is unable to perform work. This anterior tibial malfunction results in dorsal hypermobility leading to instability, which leads to increased pressure on the ligaments surrounding the joint. These ligaments, more stable plantarly than dorsally, contribute to hypermobility and lateralizing of symptoms. Lateralizing is a shifting of weight to the lateral forefoot, leading to disorders such as metatarsalgia, capsulitis, and plantar plate dysfunction.[44] A prospective, double-blinded, randomized controlled trial was performed by Faber and colleagues[57] in 2004. They compared the results of Lapidus arthrodesis vs distal first metatarsal osteotomy (Hohmann procedure) in 110 feet of patients with and without hypermobility. No difference was found between the 2 surgeries in clinical and radiographic outcomes between those with and without hypermobility with a 2-year follow-up.[57]

TISSUE STRESS THEORY

The tissue stress theory is an alternative to Root theory biomechanics that is often used in physical therapy. This theory, presented by McPoil and Hunt,[8] refers to a load-deformation curve when expressing the nature of disorders within the foot and ankle. Within this curve are 2 areas: an elastic area and a plastic area. Elastic areas represent the normal ability of soft tissues to adjust to surrounding pressures and stresses. The plastic area is where the outside limits of normal are reached and permanent, or temporary, injury will result. Application of tissue stress theory for healing ailments of the lower extremity uses 4 main steps.

> Step 1: Identify tissues that are being excessively stressed. This step is most accurately achieved by a thorough historical examination with the patient.
> Step 2: Apply controlled stress through the application of weight-bearing and non–weight-bearing tests. In addition, perform a thorough testing of muscle strength, function, and ROM abilities. Clinically, these tests include assessment of body weight and gait, as well as passive and active ROM evaluations.
> Step 3: Identify whether tissue stress is a result of excessive overloading, and then attempt to decrease it.
> Step 4: Develop a treatment protocol that effectively reduces overloading through manipulation or modification of activity levels. Institute healing of soft tissues through the application of over-the-counter or custom foot orthoses, if appropriate. Restore flexibility and muscle strength through physical therapy or stretching, allowing the individual to return to normal functional activities of daily living.[8]

SAGITTAL PLANE FACILITATION THEORY/SAGITTAL PLANE MOTION

Sagittal plane biomechanical theories have been discussed in detail in the complete works of Howard Dananberg. He describes frontal plane motion as being up to 5 times that of both frontal and transverse plane motion within the first MTPJ. For this reason, its evaluation is imperative to understanding and evaluation of first MTPJ function and disorder. Power during walking is created through the swinging limb, which allows the center of body mass to move in a forward direction over the stance phase limb, which is acting as a lever. Three rockers are described within the foot: the first is the calcaneus, the second the ankle joint, and the third the MTPJ. Sagittal plane motion can be blocked by disorders in any of these areas but a structural or functional hallux limitus results in a temporary loss in the momentum to move forward and as a result decreases the efficiency of heel-off.[58]

Functional hallux limitus is described by an event that occurs when the proximal phalanx is unable to dorsiflex on the first metatarsal. Jamming can be instantaneous (less than 100 milliseconds) and invisible to even the most trained eye. This motion was observed through the electrodynogram system, which is a segmental vertical force detector. Limitation of hallux motion may or may not be associated with pain at the joint, and other symptoms in other locations of the foot may be present as a result. When sagittal plane motion is blocked, even instantaneously, kinetic motion is trapped and must be released somewhere else. Two other joints are usually responsible for the release of this kinetic energy: the midtarsal joint and ankle joint. Sagittal plane motion is then usually taken up at the oblique axis of the midtarsal because it is the closest joint capable of sagittal plane motion, and this results in a compression of the dorsal aspect of the midtarsal joint that, with time and continued repetitive pressure, can result in collapsing of the medial arch.[22]

PREFERRED MOVEMENT PATHWAY THEORY

Nurse and Nigg[59] studied the extent that the foot responds to tactile and vibratory sensation when walking and running. They found a strong negative relationship between vibratory threshold and increased pressure under the hallux. Similar findings were noted within the heel, lateral arch, and first metatarsal head. They also found that there were individuals with more sensitivity to vibration. Data for these individuals were found to have a direct correlation to increased pressures during running, which was counterintuitive to what they believed would happen and is still unexplained.[59] The body preferentially adjusts to receive sensory input from more sensitive areas.[60] However, they believed that these findings did suggest that the body was experiencing neurologic feedback that was functioning during gait and was altering how a person walks and functions. It was suggested that consideration of these neurologic feedback systems was necessary when attempting to predict gait characteristics or implement orthotic management.[59]

    Nigg[61,62] proposed a new concept for explaining how pronation and impact forces can affect gait and potentially first ray function. The main premise of this theory is that various forces are projected on the foot during gait, in particular during the stance phase of gait. Adaptations of muscle activity then result as a secondary response to these initial forces. Every joint maintains a preferred movement response in which energy expenditure is at a minimum for motion to occur. When interventions aid in supporting this preferred movement, then energy expenditure is minimized. When interventions reduce the ability of the body to achieve this preferred movement, then energy expenditure will increase. The optimal intervention for treating disorders is one that decreases energy expenditure and optimizes muscle function. Nigg[61,62] considered that this movement control was not realigning the skeleton as was once believed, but was instead simply changing muscle function on a more localized level. However, he openly admits in his paper that this theory still requires further research and stronger evidence to refute or support his claims.[61,62]

CLINICAL EVALUATION OF THE FIRST RAY
History

As with other foot and ankle disorders, a full history and physical examination, including radiographic evaluation, should be completed. The chief complaints, and primary symptoms, of a patient with limited first ray motion are typically pain, stiffness, and inability to bend the toe. If a bump is present, this is typically at the dorsal or dorsomedial aspect of the joint. Occasionally, the main concern is the increased bulk around the joint or the bony prominence that has formed, which the patient or referring provider may mistake for a bunion deformity.

Patients may also present with secondary symptoms such as generalized foot pain or pain radiating to other parts of the foot or great toe. This may be caused by the severity of the pain or from irritation of the medial branch of the medial dorsal cutaneous nerve. Diffuse lesser metatarsalgia or sub–fifth metatarsal head pain can be presenting symptoms in the forefoot. Lateral hind foot, ankle, or knee pain can also result from a compensated gait pattern. A complete list of secondary presenting symptoms of the individual with limited first ray ROM is presented in **Box 1**.

At times, the patient may not be aware of the source of the pain and the physical examination may be required to reproduce the symptoms. Severity or intensity should be obtained, preferably with the use of a pain scale. Numerous pain scales exist, from a simple descriptive scale to a numeric or visual analog scale (VAS) or faces scale. We use the numeric scale and have the faces scale available for patients who have difficulty rating their pain numerically.

Symptoms can vary widely depending on the degree of joint deterioration, bony hypertrophy, and the compensations that may be occurring. The nature of the pain is most often described as aching but can have other qualities. Timeframes regarding symptoms should be obtained, such as duration of pain, stiffness of the joint, bony prominences, and the patient's age at the onset of these. These symptoms do not always occur together. The prominence may be seen first, followed by the stiffness, and later pain, although not always in that order (**Figs. 1** and **2**).

Some individuals present with a history of significant injury to the first metatarsophalangeal joint. Unilateral cases usually present with this scenario, whereas bilateral cases are more likely to present with a history of chronic repetitive microtrauma, with insidious onset. These presentations can also be seen in combination. The authors have treated numerous patients who presented with an acute injury as a result of forced dorsiflexion that corresponded with the onset of painful symptoms, or an exacerbation of them, but in which stiffness and bony hypertrophy had already been present. In these cases, it seems that the marginal osteophytes at the base of the proximal phalanx are fractured leading to the acute pain, as can be see in **Fig. 3**. It is possible that the acute symptoms can be improved, but not always to prior baseline levels.

Prior surgery may also contribute to the development of first MTPJ disorders. It may not be possible to know whether the original disorder was responsible for the onset of the hallux limitus/rigidus or whether it was related to the surgical intervention. For this

---

Box 1
A comprehensive list of secondary symptoms that may be noticed in the individual with first MTPJ joint limitation

Osteochondral defect first MTPJ

Callus medial or plantar HIPJ

Capsulitis sub 2

HIPJ extension

Pronation of medial column

Plantar fasciitis

Metatarsocuneiform arthritis

Subungual hematoma

Onycholysis

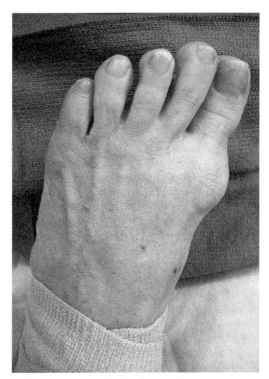

Fig. 1. The dorsomedial prominence of hallux limitus. Note flexion deformity of the hallux.

reason, when performing surgery it is beneficial to mention degenerative changes found on the operative report. In certain situations, the limitation of joint motion may not be associated with degenerative changes of the joint. In cases in which excessive scar formation or fibrosis lead to limitation of motion, the treatment may be different than that for a patient with degenerative arthritis of the joint. Iatrogenic hallux varus deformity may also have significant limitation of motion without radiographic findings

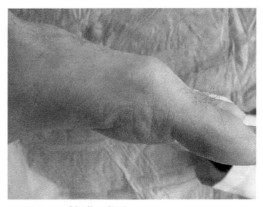

Fig. 2. The dorsal prominence of hallux limitus.

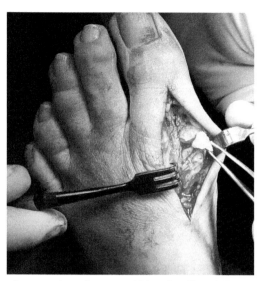

Fig. 3. Preexisting degenerative change within the first MTPJ. Note the fractured osteophyte.

of osteoarthritic changes, and correction of the deformity may be the preferred course of treatment.

It is also important to ascertain the activity level of the patient when gathering historical data. Hallux limitus or rigidus pain generally gets worse by the end of the day and with extended activity. This deterioration can be a quality-of-life issue and is often the biggest concern for the patient. Having to endure pain in order to perform desired activities, or having to avoid the activities altogether, can significantly decrease an individual's quality of life. Certain individuals require more motion of the first MTPJ secondary to the athletics or job they hold. A roofer and a dancer require more motion in the MTPJ than a 65 year old who just wants to walk for exercise.[10] Preoperative determination of the importance of these activities is important to achieve a successful treatment outcome and a satisfied patient.

Shoe gear can also contribute to the painful symptoms in the individual with limited first ray ROM. This information can provide insight into the cause of the condition. When the individual states that hiking or stiff-soled shoes decrease symptoms, pain is likely within the joint and occurs with motion of that joint. Relief when wearing deeper, wider, larger, more flexible, or open-toed shoes may indicate that the pressure to the prominence is the source of the symptoms. Determining the patient's goals and expectations with respect to shoe gear should also be discussed. A patient who is not interested in wearing high-heeled shoes, or is willing to give them up, in order to alleviate pain will likely have more treatment options than someone who needs to be in fashionable shoes. Discussing these factors with patients allows them to make more informed decisions about lifestyle changes and treatment choices.

The patient should be asked about any prior therapies and what the response to the therapy was. Information regarding accommodative orthotics and injections should be obtained. If the patient underwent surgical treatment, did the postoperative course go uneventfully or did they have any complications? How was their pain controlled? Did they have any excessive scar tissue formation?

Hallux limitus/rigidus pain can be confused with gout, particularly by those who are not specialists in the foot and ankle. Acute gout typically has a sudden onset of pain, often without a known precipitating factor, compared with hallux limitus/rigidus pain, which is more chronic and persistent, and usually not as severe.

Additional questions may be appropriate to differentiate hallux rigidus from other possible differentials such as hallux valgus, fracture, stress fracture of sesamoid or other bone, pseudogout, reactive arthritis, capsulitis, sesamoiditis, turf toe, and other systemic arthropathy.[63,64] Past medical history regarding peripheral vascular disease, neuromuscular conditions, systemic arthritic condition, osteoporosis, diabetes, smoking, immunosuppressive conditions or use of steroid medications, bleeding or coagulation disorders, medications, allergies, and family history, including problems with anesthesia, should be obtained.

Clinical Examination

Clinical examination starts with the patient's general condition. Vital signs should be obtained, including body weight. Does the patient seem well nourished? These can be important factors in determining whether the patient is a candidate for a surgical procedure and may be helpful in determining whether they are capable of following postoperative instructions.

Vascular, neurologic, dermatologic, musculoskeletal, and biomechanical examinations should be performed in each of these individuals. The vascular examination is essential to verify adequate blood flow before surgical intervention, if deemed necessary. The neurologic examination may show a positive Tinel sign in those with irritation of the digital nerve coursing over the dorsomedial prominence. Dermatologic examination shows hyperkeratosis under the HIPJ and loss of skin lines and no callus under the first MTPJ.[65] Bursitis may be noted over the dorsomedial eminence, but is more likely to be present in gout or infection. Skin and nails can also be inspected for rashes, nodules, tophi, and nail changes that may indicate the possibility of systemic causes of arthritis.[64] Musculoskeletal findings include structural deformities such as a painful dorsal prominence from bony proliferation, metatarsus primus elevatus, and hallux equinus. An associated hallux varus or valgus may be seen. Secondary compensations, as discussed earlier, in the foot and leg may also be seen. A pes planus foot type may also be observed. Dananberg[66] described lowering of the arch caused by inability of the hallux to extend.

With more severe progression of the arthritic process, ROM can be severely limited in both weight-bearing and non–weight-bearing attitudes. When compared with a more normal joint, the difference is often obvious. Similarly, more subtle cases exist. These individuals can have more limited motion on weight-bearing and full motion on non–weight-bearing examinations, with minimal change on radiographic examination. In these cases, the diagnosis of hallux limitus is more challenging. In these scenarios, we believe it most important not to rely solely on the ROM examination, but to correlate the findings of the clinical examination with the quality of motion, reproduction of symptoms, and the patient's subjective complaints in addition to radiographic presentation.

Crepitus may also be present with the ROM examination, which indicates arthritic change within the joint and possibly a loose fragment. However, lack of crepitus does not exclude the diagnosis of hallux rigidus. Fine crepitus can indicate synovitis and medium crepitus can indicate grating of roughened cartilage surfaces or bone rubbing against bone. In noninflammatory arthritic joints, more medium or course crepitus may be appreciated.[64] Pain is often present with ROM and may reproduce patient's symptoms. The central grind test involves both axial compression of the joint and rotation of the joint in the frontal plane. It can be used as a clinical indicator of articular cartilage involvement.[67,68]

Many tests are available to measure the first MTPJ and first ray ROM. The amount of motion available can vary depending on which clinical test is used. Because practitioners are often limited by time, the standard office examination involves a generalized assessment of motion by plantarflexion and dorsiflexion of the joint during closed kinetic chain. **Fig. 4** shows this technique. During this test, quality of motion, crepitus, pain, and ROM can be gathered. The overall amount of motion during gait may be overestimated with this technique, and therefore many investigators have described other techniques for determining a more accurate assessment of functional ROM of this joint. **Fig. 5** shows the technique for measuring first ray ROM. Pressure is placed in both plantar and dorsal directions on the first metatarsal head while remaining metatarsal heads are stabilized. If excessive motion is noticed in the plantar direction, a plantarflexed first ray exists. A dorsiflexed first ray also exists if excessive dorsiflexion is noticed.[11]

Testing for functional hallux limitus can be performed by testing first MTPJ ROM while preventing the first ray (metatarsal) from being able to plantarflex. Methods for testing this ROM, particularly in the dorsiflexion direction, include manual loading of the joint,[52] passive ROM while weight bearing (**Fig. 6**), active ROM while weight bearing, and the heel rise test.[32,67]

The first MTPJ of the individual with limited first ray motion may have the presence of hallux equinus, metatarsal primus elevatus, and a prominent dorsal to dorsomedial eminence. All of these can occur in isolation but usually occur in combination. Camasta[52] uses the term codependency when describing their relationship. This combination usually occurs secondary to 2 main compensations: uncompensated varus and flatfoot. Varus foot types in which the medial column does not contact the ground result in hallux gripping, which is a phenomenon in which the hallux plantarflexes in order to stabilize the medial column toward the ground. Pes planovalgus can also contribute to hallux equinus when medial structures of the foot do not adequately support the arch, resulting in a floppy or dysfunctional arch. The flexors plantarflex the hallux and, as a result, stabilize the medial column.[52]

Some discrepancy exists in the literature regarding hallux equinus and metatarsus primus elevatus. It is suggested that medial column elevation may occur primarily or secondarily. Primary elevatus can occur in a foot with forefoot varus that is uncompensated. The hallux equinus occurs as a secondary compensation within this scenario. Secondary elevatus usually occurs in a pronated foot or hypermobile foot. In this

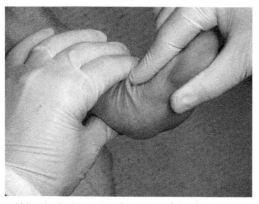

Fig. 4. Standard closed kinetic chain testing for ROM of the first MTPJ. Assessment of quality of motion, crepitus, and quantity of motion can be determined through this examination.

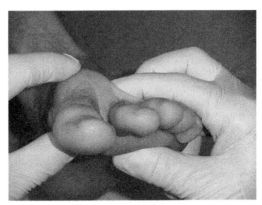

Fig. 5. Standard closed kinetic chain testing for ROM of first ray. This test is often used to evaluate for hypermobility or for plantarflexed or dorsiflexed first rays. Note the excessive dorsiflexion in this case.

situation, the hallux equinus occurs first and the metatarsal is elevated secondarily in the sagittal plane.[51] In a similar way that the Coleman block test is used to evaluate the hind foot compensation, the forefoot block test is used to assess whether a metatarsus primus elevatus is a primary or secondary disorder.[52,56] **Fig. 7** A and B show the correct method of performing the forefoot block test. If a difference in sagittal plane position of the first metatarsal is not noticed between the forefoot block and standard weight-bearing examination, then the foot has forefoot varus or spasm of the tibialis anterior tendon.[51]

Nawoczenski and colleagues[67] studied 4 clinical tests representing the spectrum of measurements typically used in the clinical setting. Two of the clinical tests, the heel rise test and the assessment of the active ROM with the subject weight bearing, were found to provide results that strongly correlated with motion of the first MTPJ during gait. In their study, the weight-bearing, active ROM test most closely matched motion during gait and was considered to be the most accurate.

First ray hypermobility should also be evaluated. The ability of the first ray to accept peak loads is the distinguishing feature as to whether hypermobility is pathologic or not. Instability is the term that is currently used to describe pathologic motion. Some patients may have inadequate first ray motion along with an efficient windlass

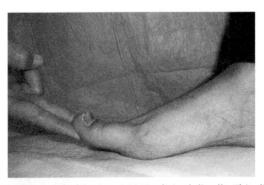

Fig. 6. Jack test. Patient is weight bearing. ROM is elicited distally. This clinical test can give the practitioner some insight into what happens during gait, but may not be the most accurate test for estimating ROM during open kinetic chain.

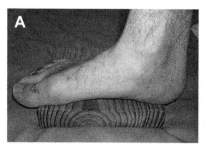 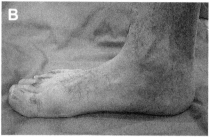

Fig. 7. (*A*) Forefoot block test is performed by having the patient weight-bearing from heel to metatarsal heads with digits dangling off the edge. (*B*) If no difference is noted in sagittal plane motion of first metatarsal between forefoot block and normal weight-bearing examination, then forefoot varus or spasm of tibialis anterior exists.

mechanism that is able to prevent disorders within the joint. The windlass mechanism is activated by dorsiflexing the hallux while the patient is weight bearing. If instability continues to exists when the windlass mechanism is activated, the joint should be considered unstable.[69,70] First and second metatarsal cuneiform joint arthritis may also be noticed in the individual with hypermobility.

Ankle equinus is associated with increased forefoot pressure as well as a decrease in the effectiveness of the peroneus longus, which may contribute to increased subtalar joint pronation and first metatarsus elevatus.[44] Charles and colleagues[71] described 2 stages of ankle equinus; a first stage in which less than 10 degrees of dorsiflexion resulted in minor increases in forefoot pressure, and a second stage in which less than 5 degrees of ankle dorsiflexion resulted in major compensations and increase in forefoot pressures.[71]

Gait analysis should be assessed for compensations of limited first ray motion, such as overloading of the lateral forefoot, early lift-off, and vertical toe-off, which is often seen with apropulsive gait in the geriatric patient. Gait is also examined for biomechanical contributions to the development of the hallux rigidus deformity.

Observation of the patient's shoe gear can also be of benefit. Signs of abnormal wear may include stretching out of the upper material or excessive wear of the sole in the region of the great toe, HIPJ, or lateral forefoot because of compensation, and a more oblique angulation at the shoe break may be seen.[72] Shoes worn to the office visit may also be an indication of the patient's typical types of shoes worn on a daily basis.[52,73] The pathologic side should always be compared with the nonpathologic side.

Diagnostic and therapeutic injections may be used in order to isolate the symptoms. These injections can be done with joint aspiration for synovial fluid analysis, if appropriate, to rule out other conditions. Synovial fluid is only diagnostic in gout, pseudogout, and infection, otherwise synovial fluid analysis can only categorize the arthritis as inflammatory or noninflammatory.[64] Screening labs may be helpful to also rule out inflammatory arthritis if suspected.

In summary, our clinical examination is a stepwise approach to assess first MTPJ and first ray ROM. The initial examination is performed with the patient sitting in passive closed kinetic chain. If ROM is significantly limited, there is no need to evaluate further. If motion is not limited with a non–weight-bearing examination, we proceed to further testing using a loading technique. Functional limitation can be assessed by loading the first ray and observing motion or by having the patient stand and perform the Jack test (see **Fig. 6**). An active ROM examination can also be performed and is the most reliable means of evaluating the motion that will occur during open kinetic chain or gait.[67]

BIOMECHANICAL RADIOGRAPHIC EVALUATION OF THE FIRST RAY

In order to evaluate biomechanical contributions to first MTPJ disorders, standard weight-bearing foot radiographs anteroposterior (AP), medial oblique, and lateral are obtained. If sesamoid disorders are found or suspected, sesamoid axial views may be obtained. Additional views such as stress dorsiflexion lateral views and radiographs while using the block tests, for assessment of the first metatarsus elevatus, can be performed. Routine assessment includes evaluation of bone density and soft tissue structures. Increases in soft tissue density surrounding a joint are consistent with joint effusion. Calcifications may also be seen. The position and foot type can be evaluated as well as the size, shape, and maturity of the bones.[74] First metatarsal and adjacent bones are assessed for shape and position. Gout may appear as increased density in the medial aspect of the first metatarsal head or as a well-defined C-shaped erosion. The contours of the joints and the internal architecture of the bones are evaluated.

Osteoarthritis is typically seen along the medial joints of the foot. Asymmetric distribution is more frequently seen; however, symmetric distribution is also seen, especially in those with systemic disease. Arthritis within other pedal joints is rare unless prior trauma contributed to its occurrence. Typical features of osteoarthritis include osteophytosis, joint space narrowing, subchondral sclerosis, subchondral cyst formation, and loose osseous body.[74]

Hypertrophy and arthritic changes of the sesamoids may also be seen. Osteopenia of the sesamoids may be noted, in particular if there is disuse, as can be seen with metatarsus primus elevatus. As the sesamoids become completely fused to the plantar metatarsal head, hallux rigidus ensues. Proximal migration of the sesamoids will also occur with a contracted FHB muscle, as can be seen with hallux equinus.[52]

Metatarsus elevatus is not necessarily associated with limited first ray motion because elevation can be seen even in the absence of symptoms. Average values between the cortices of metatarsals 1 and 2 can be up to 7 mm.[55] **Fig. 8** shows an individual with metatarsus primus elevatus. Bryant and colleagues[54] found a significant association between the hallux interphalangeal angle (HIPA) and hallux limitus. A significant correlation between increased metatarsal width, positive first metatarsal protrusion, metatarsus adductus and the development of a bunion was also found.

Lateral intermetatarsal angle was studied by Bryant and colleagues[75] in 2001. This angle comprises the angular divergence of metatarsal cortices 1 and 2 and is viewed on lateral radiograph. They found a small but significant difference in those with hallux limitus compared with their normal population. The average was found to be

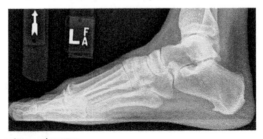

Fig. 8. Metatarsus primus elevatus.

1.02 degrees within the normal population, and 3.22 degrees was the average in those with hallux limitus.[75] A similar means of evaluation was performed by Camasta and Cicchinelli and colleagues and was found to be both reproducible and accurate.[52,76]

Hypermobility can also be evaluated on radiograph. Myerson and Badekas[56] describe a technique in which AP views are evaluated with and without strapping of the forefoot. Subjective values were not given to describe what was considered hypermobile and what was not. They also refer to increased diastasis between first and second metatarsal and the second cuneiform as a sign of hypermobility.[56]

A variety of classification systems for hallux limitus/rigidus have been described in the literature. Regnauld[77] graded findings ranging from grade I to grade III, and Hanft and colleagues[78] expanded this to include grades IIB and IIIB.

SUMMARY

Evaluation of the first ray is complex and requires an understanding of not only how the first ray functions but also how the remainder of the foot contributes to the function of the first ray. The science of first ray function was initiated by many of the pioneers such as Morton, Root, Hicks, Lapidus, and continues to evolve through the work of many other biomechanical experts such as Kirby, Dananberg, Christensen, Nigg, Mann, and Shereff. Continued study of the first ray and the shift toward evidence-based medicine has led to a more complete understanding of foot function and first ray function.

The specialist evaluating the foot for biomechanical deformities and associated pathologies must use numerous diagnostic tools in the workup. In some cases, the decision making may be straightforward because the arthritic findings may be severe on clinical and radiographic examination. In these cases, there may not be the need for more extensive examination. At other times, the findings are subtle and numerous tools may be necessary to gain a full appreciation of the biomechanics at play and their effect on the first MTPJ. We have outlined several techniques that are at our disposal when evaluating these patients and clinicians must use their best judgment as to which of these tests are appropriate for a particular situation. It would not be practical to use all of these clinical or radiographic tools in every situation. Functional hallux limitus may present more subtly and may present a greater clinical challenge to the specialist in both workup and treatment. The tools outlined here can help guide the practitioner treating these conditions. Incorporation of some of these clinical tests can allow a more thorough clinical assessment and more optimal outcomes for our patients.

REFERENCES

1. Bojsen-Moller F. Calcaneocuboid joint and stability of the longitudinal arch of the foot at high and low gear push off. J Anat 1979;129(Pt 1):165–76.
2. Hicks JH. The mechanics of the foot. I. The joints. J Anat 1953;87(4):345–57.
3. Harris RI, Beath T. The short first metatarsal; its incidence and clinical significance. J Bone Joint Surg Am 1949;31(3):553–65.
4. Glasoe WM, Coughlin MJ. A critical analysis of Dudley Morton's concept of disordered foot function. J Foot Ankle Surg 2006;45(3):147–55.
5. Rodgers MM, Cavanagh PR. Pressure distribution in Morton's foot structure. Med Sci Sports Exerc 1989;21(1):23–8.
6. Skliar JD. Critique of podiatric biomechanics by William Eric Lee, DPM. Clin Podiatr Med Surg 2001;18(4):685–90, vi.

7. Lee WE. Podiatric biomechanics. An historical appraisal and discussion of the Root model as a clinical system of approach in the present context of theoretical uncertainty. Clin Podiatr Med Surg 2001;18(4):555–684 [discussion: 685–90], v.

8. McPoil TG, Hunt GC. Evaluation and management of foot and ankle disorders: present problems and future directions. J Orthop Sports Phys Ther 1995;21(6): 381–8.

9. Valmassey R. Clinical biomechanics of the lower extremities. St Louis: Mosby-Year Book; 1996.

10. Hetherington VJ, Carnett J, Patterson BA. Motion of the first metatarsophalangeal joint. J Foot Surg 1989;28(1):13–9.

11. Root ML, Orien WP, Weed JH. Clinical biomechanics, vol. 2. Los Angeles (CA): Clinical Biomechanics Corporation; 1977.

12. Roukis TS, Landsman AS. Hypermobility of the first ray: a critical review of the literature. J Foot Ankle Surg 2003;42(6):377–90.

13. Roukis TS, Scherer PR, Anderson CF. Position of the first ray and motion of the first metatarsophalangeal joint. J Am Podiatr Med Assoc 1996;86(11):538–46.

14. Boyd N, Brock H, Meier A, et al. Extensor hallucis capsularis: frequency and identification on MRI. Foot Ankle Int 2006;27(3):181–4.

15. McCarthy DJ. The surgical anatomy of the first ray. Part I: the distal segment. J Am Podiatry Assoc 1983;73(3):111–21.

16. Johnson CH, Christensen JC. Biomechanics of the first ray. Part I. The effects of peroneus longus function: a three-dimensional kinematic study on a cadaver model. J Foot Ankle Surg 1999;38(5):313–21.

17. Johnson CH, Christensen JC. Biomechanics of the first ray part V: the effect of equinus deformity. A 3-dimensional kinematic study on a cadaver model. J Foot Ankle Surg 2005;44(2):114–20.

18. Basmajian JV, Bentzon JW. An electromyographic study of certain muscles of the leg and foot in the standing position. Surg Gynecol Obstet 1954;98(6): 662–6.

19. McCarthy DJ. The surgical anatomy of the first ray. Part II: the proximal segment. J Am Podiatry Assoc 1983;73(5):244–55.

20. Mizel MS. The role of the plantar first metatarsal first cuneiform ligament in weightbearing on the first metatarsal. Foot Ankle 1993;14(2):82–4.

21. Ebisui JM. The first ray axis and the first metatarsophalangeal joint: an anatomical and pathomechanical study. J Am Podiatry Assoc 1968;58(4):160–8.

22. Dananberg HJ. Functional hallux limitus and its relationship to gait efficiency. J Am Podiatr Med Assoc 1986;76(11):648–52.

23. Perez HR, Reber LK, Christensen JC. The effect of frontal plane position on first ray motion: forefoot locking mechanism. Foot Ankle Int 2008;29(1):72–6.

24. Hiss L. Foot disorders. Los Angeles (CA): Los Angeles University Press; 1937.

25. Kelikian H. Structural alteration. In: Hallux valgus, allied deformities of the foot and metatarsalgia. Philadelphia: WB Saunders; 1965.

26. Joseph J. Great toe motion in men. J Bone Joint Surg 1954;36B:450.

27. Mann RA, Hagy JL. The function of the toes in walking, jogging and running. Clin Orthop Relat Res 1979;(142):24–9.

28. Bojsen-Moller F, Lamoreux L. Significance of free-dorsiflexion of the toes in walking. Acta Orthop Scand 1979;50(4):471–9.

29. Shereff MJ, Bejjani FJ, Kummer FJ. Kinematics of the first metatarsophalangeal joint. J Bone Joint Surg 1986;68:392–8.

30. Buell T, Green DR, Risser J. Measurement of the first metatarsophalangeal joint range of motion. J Am Podiatr Med Assoc 1988;78(9):439–48.

31. Hetherington VJ, Johnson RE, Albritton JS. Necessary dorsiflexion of the first metatarsophalangeal joint during gait. J Foot Surg 1990;29(3):218–22.
32. Hopson MM, McPoil TG, Cornwall MW. Motion of the first metatarsophalangeal joint. Reliability and validity of four measurement techniques. J Am Podiatr Med Assoc 1995;85(4):198–204.
33. Zammit GV, Menz HB, Munteanu SE, et al. Plantar pressure distribution in older people with osteoarthritis of the first metatarsophalangeal joint (hallux limitus/rigidus). J Orthop Res 2008;26(12):1665–9.
34. Brahm SM. Shape of the first metatarsal head in hallux rigidus and hallux valgus. J Am Podiatr Med Assoc 1988;78(6):300–4.
35. Kilmartin TE, Wallace WA. First metatarsal head shape in juvenile hallux abducto valgus. J Foot Surg 1991;30(5):506–8.
36. Mancuso JE, Abramow SP, Landsman MJ, et al. The zero-plus first metatarsal and its relationship to bunion deformity. J Foot Ankle Surg 2003;42(6): 319–26.
37. Okuda R, Kinoshita M, Yasuda T, et al. The shape of the lateral edge of the first metatarsal head as a risk factor for recurrence of hallux valgus. J Bone Joint Surg Am 2007;89(10):2163–72.
38. Schweitzer ME, Maheshwari S, Shabshin N. Hallux valgus and hallux rigidus: MRI findings. Clin Imaging 1999;23(6):397–402.
39. Coughlin MJ, Shurnas PS. Hallux rigidus. Grading and long-term results of operative treatment. J Bone Joint Surg Am 2003;85(11):2072–88.
40. Perez HR, Reber LK, Christensen JC. Effects on the metatarsophalangeal joint after simulated first tarsometatarsal joint arthrodesis. J Foot Ankle Surg 2007; 46(4):242–7.
41. Hicks JH. The mechanics of the foot. II. The plantar aponeurosis and the arch. J Anat 1954;88(1):25–30.
42. Kappel-Bargas A, Woolf RD, Cornwall MW, et al. The windlass mechanism during normal walking and passive first metatarsalphalangeal joint extension. Clin Biomech (Bristol, Avon) Apr 1998;13(3):190–4.
43. Aquino A, Payne C. Function of the windlass mechanism in excessively pronated feet. J Am Podiatr Med Assoc 2001;91(5):245–50.
44. Rush SM, Christensen JC, Johnson CH. Biomechanics of the first ray. Part II: metatarsus primus varus as a cause of hypermobility. A three-dimensional kinematic analysis in a cadaver model. J Foot Ankle Surg 2000;39(2):68–77.
45. Fuller EA. The windlass mechanism of the foot. A mechanical model to explain pathology. J Am Podiatr Med Assoc 2000;90(1):35–46.
46. D'Ambrogi E, Giacomozzi C, Macellari V, et al. Abnormal foot function in diabetic patients: the altered onset of Windlass mechanism. Diabet Med 2005;22(12): 1713–9.
47. Roling BA, Christensen JC, Johnson CH. Biomechanics of the first ray. Part IV: the effect of selected medial column arthrodeses. A three-dimensional kinematic analysis in a cadaver model. J Foot Ankle Surg 2002;41(5):278–85.
48. Faber FW, Kleinrensink GJ, Verhoog MW, et al. Mobility of the first tarsometatarsal joint in relation to hallux valgus deformity: anatomical and biomechanical aspects. Foot Ankle Int 1999;20(10):651–6.
49. Avino A, Patel S, Hamilton GA, et al. The effect of the Lapidus arthrodesis on the medial longitudinal arch: a radiographic review. J Foot Ankle Surg 2008;47(6): 510–4.
50. Phillips RD, Law EA, Ward ED. Functional motion of the medial column joints of the foot during propulsion. J Am Podiatr Med Assoc 1996;86(10):474–86.

51. Banks AS, Downey MS, Martin DE, et al. McGlamry's Comprehensive textbook of foot and ankle surgery, vol. 1. 3rd edition. Philadelphia: Lippincott Williams & Wilkins; 2001.
52. Camasta CA. Hallux limitus and hallux rigidus. Clinical examination, radiographic findings, and natural history. Clin Podiatr Med Surg 1996;13(3):423–48.
53. Youngswick FD. Modifications of the Austin bunionectomy for treatment of metatarsus primus elevatus associated with hallux limitus. J Foot Surg 1982;21(2):114–6.
54. Bryant A, Tinley P, Singer K. A comparison of radiographic measurements in normal, hallux valgus, and hallux limitus feet. J Foot Ankle Surg 2000;39(1):39–43.
55. Meyer JO, Nishon LR, Weiss L, et al. Metatarsus primus elevatus and the etiology of hallux rigidus. J Foot Surg 1987;26(3):237–41.
56. Myerson MS, Badekas A. Hypermobility of the first ray. Foot Ankle Clin 2000;5(3):469–84.
57. Faber FW, Mulder PG, Verhaar JA. Role of first ray hypermobility in the outcome of the Hohmann and the Lapidus procedure. A prospective, randomized trial involving one hundred and one feet. J Bone Joint Surg Am 2004;86(3):486–95.
58. Dananberg HJ. Sagittal plane biomechanics. American Diabetes Association. J Am Podiatr Med Assoc 2000;90(1):47–50.
59. Nurse MA, Nigg BM. Quantifying a relationship between tactile and vibration sensitivity of the human foot with plantar pressure distributions during gait. Clin Biomech (Bristol, Avon) 1999;14(9):667–72.
60. Nurse MA, Nigg BM. The effect of changes in foot sensation on plantar pressure and muscle activity. Clin Biomech (Bristol, Avon) 2001;16(9):719–27.
61. Nigg BM. The role of impact forces and foot pronation: a new paradigm. Clin J Sport Med 2001;11(1):2–9.
62. Nigg BM, Nurse MA, Stefanyshyn DJ. Shoe inserts and orthotics for sport and physical activities. Med Sci Sports Exerc 1999;31(Suppl 7):S421–8.
63. Logan D, McKee PJ. Poststreptococcal reactive arthritis. J Am Podiatr Med Assoc 2006;96(4):362–6.
64. Klippel JH, Stone JH, Crofford LJ, et al. Primer on the rheumatic diseases. 13th edition. New York (NY): Springer-Verlag; 2008.
65. Lapidus PW. Dorsal bunion: its mechanics and operative correction. J Bone Joint Surg 1940;22:627–37.
66. Dananberg HJ. Gait style as an etiology to chronic postural pain. Part I. Functional hallux limitus. J Am Podiatr Med Assoc 1993;83(8):433–41.
67. Nawoczenski DA, Baumhauer JF, Umberger BR. Relationship between clinical measurements and motion of the first metatarsophalangeal joint during gait. J Bone Joint Surg Am 1999;81:370–6.
68. Baumhauer JF. Dorsal cheilectomy of the first metatarsophalangeal joint in the treatment of hallux rigidus. Oper Tech Orthop 1999;9(1):26–32.
69. Christensen JC, Jennings MM. Normal and abnormal function of the first ray. Clin Podiatr Med Surg 2009;26(3):355–71, Table of Contents.
70. Coughlin MJ, Smith BW. Hallux valgus and first ray mobility. Surgical technique. J Bone Joint Surg Am 2008;90(Suppl 2 Pt 2):153–70.
71. Charles J, Scutter SD, Buckley J. Static ankle joint equinus: toward a standard definition and diagnosis. J Am Podiatr Med Assoc 2010;100(3):195–203.
72. Bingold AC, Collins DH. Hallux rigidus. J Bone Joint Surg Br 1950;32(2):214–22.
73. Alexander IJ. The foot examination and diagnosis. 2nd edition. New York: Churchill Livingstone Inc; 1997.
74. Christman RA. Foot and Ankle Radiology. St Louis: Elsevier Health Sciences; 2003.

75. Bryant A, Mahoney B, Tinley P. Lateral intermetatarsal angle: a useful measurement of metatarsus primus elevatus? J Am Podiatr Med Assoc 2001;91(5):251–4.
76. Cicchinelli LD, Camasta CA, McGlamry ED. Iatrogenic metatarsus primus elevatus. Etiology, evaluation, and surgical management. J Am Podiatr Med Assoc 1997;87(4):165–77.
77. Regnauld B, editor. The foot: Pathology, aetiology, seminology, clinical investigation and treatment. New York: Springer-Verlag; 1986.
78. Hanft JR, Mason ET, Landsman AS, et al. A new radiographic classification for hallux limitus. J Foot Ankle Surg 1993;32(4):397–404.

Sesamoid Disorders of the First Metatarsophalangeal Joint

Allan Boike, DPM[e], Molly Schnirring-Judge, DPM[a,b,c,d],*,
Sean McMillin, DPM[f]

KEYWORDS

• Sesamoids • Feet • First metatarsophalangeal joint • Disorders

The sesamoids of the feet were named by Galen circa 180 CE because of their resemblance to sesame seeds. These tiny bones were believed by the ancient Hebrews to be indestructible and therefore the housing for the soul after death, which would ultimately be resurrected on the Day of Judgment.[1] However, the sesamoid complex, which transmits 50% of body weight and more than 300% during push-off, is not invincible and is susceptible to numerous pathologies.[2,3] These pathologies include sesamoiditis, stress fracture, avascular necrosis, osteochondral fractures, and chondromalacia, and are secondary to these large weight-bearing loads. This article discusses sesamoid conditions and their relationship with hallux limitus, and reviews the conditions that predispose the first metatarsophalangeal joint (MPJ) to osteoarthritic changes.

There is much debate regarding the causes of hallux limitus and rigidus and the role of the sesamoids in precipitating the decreased range of motion of the first MPJ has been considered in some detail. Typically, little is done to the sesamoids at the time of surgical treatment of the hallux limitus deformity. This article reviews the recent

[a] Cleveland Clinic Foundation- Kaiser Permanente Podiatric Surgical Residency Program, 10 Severence Circle, Cleveland Heights, OH 44070, USA
[b] Ohio University, Firelands Regional Medical Center, Residency Training Program, 111 Hayes Avenue, Sandusky, OH 44870, USA
[c] Graduate Medical Education, Mercy Health Partners, Toledo, OH, USA
[d] Private Practice, North West Ohio Foot and Ankle Institute, LLC, 530 Washington Street, Port Clinton, OH 43452, USA
[e] Foot and Ankle Center, Orthopaedic and Rheumatologic Institute, Cleveland Clinic, Cleveland, Ohio
[f] Cleveland Clinic/Kaiser Permanente, Department of Orthopaedics Podiatric Residency Training Program, Cleveland, Ohio
* Corresponding author. Cleveland Clinic Foundation- Kaiser Permanente Podiatric Surgical Residency Program, 10 Severence Circle, Cleveland Heights, OH 44070.
E-mail address: mjudgemolly@aim.com

Clin Podiatr Med Surg 28 (2011) 269–285
doi:10.1016/j.cpm.2011.03.006
0891-8422/11/$ – see front matter © 2011 Elsevier Inc. All rights reserved.

literature of sesamoid disorders and, more specifically, their role in hallux limitus. Potential treatment options are also discussed.

ANATOMY

The sesamoids are located centrally and plantar to the first metatarsal head where they are imbedded within the plantar plate. There are 3 sesamoids associated with the great toe joint; 2 are considered constant and lie beneath the first metatarsal head, and the third, referred to as inconstant, when present develops inferior to the hallux interphalangeal joint (HIPJ). These bones may be semiovoid, bean shaped, or circular and so are considered variable in morphology. The 2 sesamoids of the first MPJ are not typically equal in size. The tibial sesamoid is larger, ovoid, and elongated, and is encased within the medial head of the flexor hallucis brevis (FHB) tendon. The smaller fibular sesamoid is smaller and more circular and is surrounded by the lateral head of the FHB tendon. The larger size of the tibial sesamoid bears more weight than the fibular sesamoid and is believed to predispose the medial sesamoid to more pathology. Portions of the adductor and abductor hallucis tendons also insert on the sesamoids. The sesamoids are suspended by a medial and lateral sesamoidal ligament that extends from the metatarsal head and inserts on the medial portion of the tibial sesamoid and lateral portion of the fibular sesamoid. This ligamentous stirrup-type arrangement about the sesamoid apparatus contributes to the plantar plate of the first MTPJ; a structure understood to be vital to the gliding function of the joint. An additional ligamentous attachment includes the deep transverse intermetatarsal ligament (DTIL) extending from the fibular sesamoid to the neck of the second metatarsal as well as an intersesamoidal ligament that serves as an attachment between the sesamoids and contributes to the plantar plate.[1,2,4,5]

The function of the sesamoids is to absorb and disperse weight bearing from the metatarsal head. This function in turn provides protection to the flexor hallucis longus (FHL) tendon.[4,6] The sesamoids increase the moment arm of the flexors, increasing their power and supplementing the mechanical advantage of 1st MTPJ motion. The sesamoids are invested within the FHB tendons and function to absorb shock and enhance the gliding function of the MTPJ.[4]

Understanding the arterial supply to the sesamoids is important to investigating sesamoid injury, understanding healing and allows for more accurate prognostication regarding surgical outcomes. Each sesamoid has been shown to receive its own individual artery for nutrition, but may have 2 or 3. Blood supply stems from the medial plantar artery (25%), the plantar arch (25%), or from both sources (50%).[2,4] Both sesamoids receive blood supply from proximal and plantar sources, but are less well vascularized distally. The proximal supply enters through the FHB insertion, and plantarly via midline capsular attachments. The more sparse distal supply comes from the capsule and may help explain some disorders such as osteonecrosis or nonunion of fractures (**Fig. 1**).[1,2] Because of the predominately plantar vascular supply, incisional approaches are safer from the dorsum or medial approach.[4]

Ossification of the sesamoids occurs between the ages of 7 and 10 years, beginning usually with the fibular sesamoid followed by the tibial sesamoid.[5] Agenesis or congenital absence of the sesamoids is rare. There are typically multiple ossification centers, which may result in bipartite sesamoids caused by incomplete fusion of these 2 centers. The tibial sesamoid is bipartite in approximately 10% of the population (**Fig. 2**A, B), whereas the fibular sesamoid is rarely bipartite. In patients who have a bipartite tibial sesamoid, 25% have the bilateral condition.[2,4] Weil and Hill[7] reported a statistically significant correlation between the incidence of a bipartite tibial

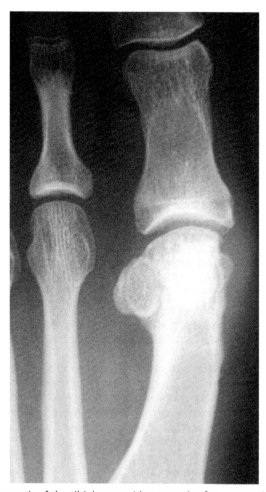

Fig. 1. Avascular necrosis of the tibial sesamoid as a result of an aggressive debridement of the medial eminence to reduce a bunion deformity. Note the sclerotic appearance of the sesamoid bone and the irregular residual medial border of the metatarsal head and neck as evidence of an aggressive eminence resection. The vascular supply to the sesamoids is at risk whenever surgical intervention for reduction of the bunion deformity is pursued.

sesamoid and hallux valgus deformity, hypothesizing that the bipartite tibial sesamoid causes an imbalance in the intrinsic musculature.

CLINICAL FINDINGS

Sesamoid disorders account for 9% of foot and ankle injuries and 1.2% of running injuries.[2] Although any one can suffer from a sesamoid disorder, chronic sesamoid afflictions seem to occur more frequently in active patient populations. The pain associated with sesamoid disorders is variable and can range from generalized joint pain or capsulitis of the first MPJ to pain localized to the affected sesamoid or the sesamoid apparatus plantarly. The pain may be constant or simply aggravated by weight-bearing activity. A chief complaint of pain around the big toe or the sensation of a snapping about the joint after running can be the harbinger of sesamoid

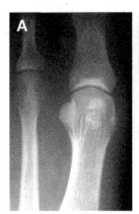
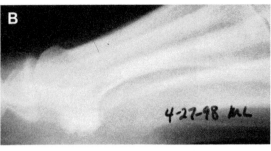

Fig. 2. (*A*) Bipartite tibial sesamoid on plain film dorsal plantar projection. Associated here with a short first ray segment and functional hallux limitus, it is easy to appreciate that the tibial sesamoid is in 2 pieces with a well-circumscribed erosion within its most proximal lateral pole. The distal pole appears almost crescent in shape. (*B*) The bifid appearance can be elucidated from this view; however, given the overlap with the fibular sesamoid, the dorsal plantar view remains the optimal projection to assess this morphology.

dysfunction. Generally, pain is expressed during the final stage of stance phase when the hallux is extended. Trauma, a change in activity or an increase in typical activity may
precede an acute fracture or stress fracture. Burning, radiating, or pins-and-needles sensation may indicate neuritis incited by edema, inflammation, or by a displaced fracture.[5] The differential diagnosis associated with sesamoid disorders includes, but is not limited to, acute fracture, osteochondritis, repetitive stress injury, osteoarthritis (**Fig. 3**), sesamoiditis (acute, subacute or chronic), infection, nerve impingement, and intractable plantar keratoses.[1]

The physical examination often reveals pain with end range of motion of the first MTPJ with dorsiflexion. Evidence of edema, loss of active and passive dorsiflexion, and weakness with plantar flexion may be associated with sesamoid disorders. Direct palpation plantarly and translocating the sesamoids distally usually elicits pain as well. A reactive synovitis or capsulitis can be identified with pain around the periphery of the joint. The clinical examination should include a stance evaluation to identify structural deformity such as pes cavus. Since this foot type is associated with a plantar flexed 1st ray sesamoiditis and metatarsalagia are hallmark for this pateint subset. This structural imbalance increases stress and load on the sesamoid apparatus and can elicit symptoms such as stress reactions, intractable plantar keratosis, or sesamoid stress fracture. The medial eminence of the metatarsal head can be percussed to determine whether there is reproducible burning pain or numbness indicating an inflamed plantar digital nerve.[4,5] Given the myriad of disorders that may affect the first MTPJ, sesamoid disorders are often a diagnosis of exclusion and so it is important to evaluate this condition thoroughly and follow the clinical course closely. Although the pain of sesamoiditis (see **Fig. 3**) and avascular necrosis (AVN) of the sesamoid (see **Fig. 1**) may be similar, the prognosis for these conditions is very different. The tibial sesamoid is more commonly associated with fracture due to its increased load bearing in stance as compared to the fibular sesamoid. When sub sesamoid pain is associated with a fragmented sesamoid with irregular borders or separation of these parts the provisional diagnosis is sesamoid fracture.

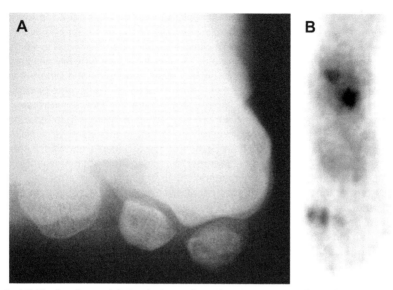

Fig. 3. (*A*) The forefoot axial view is the preferred projection to evaluate the sesamoid apparatus and the condition of the sesamoid articulations. Here there are numerous cysts within both sesamoids, whereas the morphology of the cristae and the integrity of the sesamoid joint spaces remains intact. It is the entire metatarsal head that is shifted into valgus, maintaining a congruous relationship between the sesamoids and the crista. This condition is a common finding in association with hallux abducto valgus, as opposed to that seen with hallux limitus, in which the sesamoid degeneration is best appreciated in this view. (*B*) This is the 3rd phase of a triphasic bone scan in a case of sesamoiditis. Notice that the fibular sesamoid appears larger and is more ovoid than the well rounded tibial sesamoid in this case. Focal symptomatology is evident upon direct palpation of the sesamoid apparatus; worse beneath the fibular sesamoid in this 40-year old athlete.

RADIOGRAPHIC EVALUATION AND IMAGING

Generally, weight-bearing radiographs are obtained. The lateral radiograph provides little insight into the condition. An anteroposterior view can sometimes illustrate a bipartite sesamoid or fractures. A medial oblique view is obtained to stress the tibial sesamoid, whereas a lateral oblique view stresses the fibular sesamoid. A sesamoid axial view allows inspection of the sesamoids, cristae, and the position of the sesamoidal apparatus (see **Fig. 3**A).[3–5]

When plain radiographs do not suggest deformity or injury ancillary imaging may be warranted. It is understood that the symptoms of a stress fracture in general precede radiographic changes and so nuclear medicine imaging, specifically the 99mTc-MDP scan is reliable in identifying the hyperemia of this condition in advance. In general bone scans have a high sensitivity but low specificity in determining musculoskeletal disease. A dorsal plantar view or posteroanterior bone scan is recommended to distinguish sesamoid disorders from first MTPJ disorders, which can be obstructed in an anteroposterior scan (**Fig. 3**).[5] Oblique views of the forefoot best separate the sesamoid from the metatarsal bone and reveal isolated hyperemia within the sesamoid bones using intravenous 99m Tc-methylene diphosphonate (99mTc-MDP). It is also wise to compare a scan of the afflicted foot with the contralateral foot. An increase in uptake in the affected foot compared with the contralateral foot is significant for pathology and suggests injury or active remodeling of bone resulting in hyperemia.[3]

Although localized sub–first MTPJ pain associated with a sesamoid bone found on plain radiographs to be in two pieces is clinically diagnostic of a fractured sesamoid, a bone scan can be useful when there is a clinical question between what is a bipartite sesamoid and what is a fractured sesamoid. The acute fracture typically has irregular and jagged borders while more chronic inflammatory conditions of a bipartite sesamoid present with rounded margins and well defined borders. Transverse plane separation of the parts or comminution is also suggestive of fracture. Further if the separation of the fragments is large it is more suggestive of fracture than other conditions and contralateral views are particularly important in this instance. Chisin and colleagues[8] found that 26% to 29% of asymptomatic patients showed increased uptake in the sesamoid region, so nuclear medicine imaging is not necessarily useful in the evaluation of the asymptomatic condition.

A computerized tomography (CT) scan can assist the clinician in diagnosing a stress fracture or nonunion, and can delineate posttraumatic changes compared with the contralateral part.[2,4,5] Magnetic resonance imaging (MRI) offers little in the direct diagnosis of sesamoid disorders, but does provide clues to surrounding first MPJ disorders including flexor hallucis tendonitis, plantar plate disorders, osteochondral injury, or gout.[2] This modality may be useful if attempting to diagnose osteomyelitis of the sesamoid.[3,5] The senior author has extensive experience with nuclear medicine imaging (NMI) for the evaluation of foot and ankle disorders and has found it especially powerful when investigating musculoskeletal disorders. Even the small and well-defined structures of the forefoot can be resolved using this modality and, in osteomyelitis, this modality is particularly helpful (**Figs. 3**A and **4**C).

SESAMOIDITIS

Sesamoiditis is a generalized term for a painful inflammatory condition associated with a sesamoid complex devoid of radiographic changes. Teens and young adults have a higher predilection for this disorder. Factors that increase susceptibility include a plantar flexed first ray, asymmetry in size, condylar malformation, rotational malalignment, and symmetric enlargement. Physical examination can reveal pain with direct palpation or passive distal push on the sesamoid apparatus, passive dorsiflexion of the hallux, and crepitus along the distal course of the FHL. There may be edema, bursal thickening, and inflammation plantarly (**Fig. 5**).[2,4,5]

Conservative treatment for chronic sesamoiditis and most other sesamoid disorders includes rest, ice, nonsteroidal anti-inflammatory medications, and custom modified orthoses. These conditions are often caused by repetitive stress, and correcting any abnormal biomechanical influences is the key to long-term success. This correction can be done in a variety of ways including activity modification, custom modified orthoses, gel inserts under the sesamoids, a metatarsal bar, OrthoWedge shoe, or modified cast immobilization for stress fractures or acute fractures. Bone stimulation can also be used to compliment other conservative treatments when a delayed union or nonunion of sesamoid fracture is suspected. Adjusting custom orthotics to include a Morton extension may be effective, as well as using a carbon fiber forefoot plate to restrict forefoot motion.[2,4,5]

Surgical treatment of recalcitrant disorders has been varied. Before the 1980s, excision was the primary treatment.[2] In 1914, Speed recommended that if 1 sesamoid is excised, then the other should be removed as well to prevent increased pressure on the lone sesamoid.[8] Subsequently, this led to an increased incidence of cock-up deformity of the hallux and is no longer recommended. However singular excision was advocated for conditions such as displaced and nondisplaced fractures,

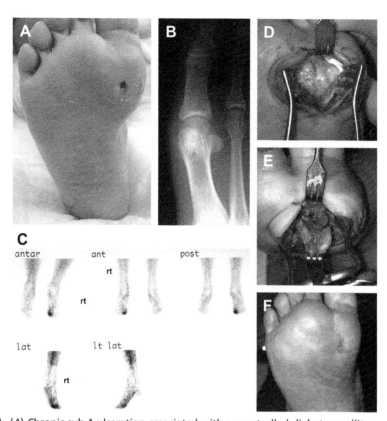

Fig. 4. (*A*) Chronic sub 1 ulceration associated with uncontrolled diabetes mellitus, peripheral vascular disease, and peripheral neuropathy. The primary care physician had been treating sesamoiditis for 4 weeks until the ulceration developed. This ulceration was hardly noticed by the patient and, were it not for the drainage noted on her socks, she may never have reported this condition. She had been treated with 2 months of oral antibiotics before referral to a foot and ankle specialist. (*B*) In this plain film, the tibial sesamoid is found to be degenerate with a squared-off medial segment and a multipartite morphology discerned within the lateral half of the bone, reflective of chronic disease. The fibular sesamoid does not appear to be affected by the degenerative process. (*C*) This example of NMI using 99mTc-monoclonal antibody imaging reveals an infectious process well localized to the plantar aspect of the first MPJ without evidence of extension into the hallux. Given the underlying peripheral vascular disease, it is easy to appreciate that the vascular tree is competent to provide isotope to the entire lower extremity without exception. (*D*) Squaring of the tibial sesamoid and multipartite lateral half of that bone correlates well with that noted in the plain film (*B*). (*E*) Underlying the sesamoid apparatus, the inferior aspect of the first metatarsal head can be appreciated and is found to be degenerate in this region. Excision of the tibial sesamoid and local debridement of the affected inferior surface of the metatarsal head is complimented by intravenous antibiotic therapy for 3-weeks' duration. This treatment proved to be curative with the benefit of long-term management using custom-molded diabetic insoles and firm-soled, extra-depth shoe gear. (*F*) Clinical appearance 5 months status after delayed primary closure followed by 3 weeks of intravenous vancomycin adjusted for renal impairment. Long-term management is supplemented by routine follow-up for palliative care of residual keratotic overgrowth. Serologic studies returned to normal baseline parameters immediately after the delayed primary closure and updated serologic testing remains within normal limits more than 4 months after the antibiotic therapy was discontinued.

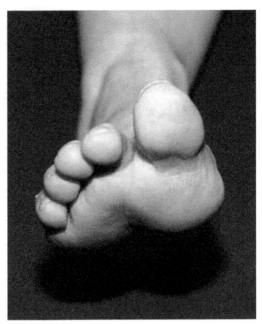

Fig. 5. The clinical appearance of the combination of an inflamed bursal projection and sesamoiditis results in a profound soft tissue enlargement beneath the metatarsal head accentuating the presence of the plantar flexed first ray in this patient.

sesamoiditis or osteochondritis that does not resolve with 6 months of conservative management, and osteomyelitis.[8] Although isolated sesamoid resection can prove definitive, this procedure is has potential complications. Removing the fibular sesamoid is associated with an increased incidence of hallux varus, whereas removing a tibial sesamoid can worsen a hallux valgus deformity. Excision of either sesamoid can increase the stress or pressure on the metatarsal head and FHL tendon producing localized disorders.[2] To avoid these complications, alternate surgical procedures have been suggested. Curettage with grafting has been reported for nonunion and AVN.[2] Aquino and colleagues[9] reported an 89% subjective success of plantar shaving for intractable plantar keratosis. Open reduction and internal fixation with 2.0-mm screws has been described for displaced acute fractures as well as percutaneous internal fixation for nondisplaced fractures using cannulated screws.[2] Based upon predictable ill effects, sesamoid excision is reserved as a last ditch effort and often precedes a joint destructive procedure.

The Procedure: Isolated Sesamoid Excision

Four techniques are used depending on the disorder, and include either an intra-articular medial, extra-articular medial, standard dorsolateral, or plantar approach.

An intra-articular medial approach provides the advantage of visualizing and inspecting the MTPJ. This approach begins with a 3-cm to 4-cm incision medially extending from the proximal flare of the metatarsal head to the midshaft of the proximal phalanx. Care is taken to protect the medial plantar nerve in this dissection. A linear capsulotomy is performed just inferior to the abductor hallucis. The plantar capsule, consisting of the retinaculum and metatarsosesamoid ligament can be incised to allow visualization of the tibial sesamoid articular surface as well as the metatarsal head and proximal phalangeal base. At this point, any hypertrophic syno-vitis can be resected, intersesamoidal ligament tears can be identified, and the condi-tion of the FHL tendon can be assessed. Using this incision, autogenous bone graft could be harvested from the distal portion of the first metatarsal if desired. A beaver blade is commonly used to sharply circumscribe the sesamoids to shell them out of their tendinous investments. Closure consists of 2-0 absorbable suture for plantar capsule repair, 3-0 absorbable suture for reapproximation of the medial capsular inci-sion, and the surgeon's preference thereafter for the subsequent layered closure.[2,5]

The extra-articular medial approach is useful for plantar shaving of a hypertrophic or prominent sesamoid or for grafting of a nonunion without an articular step-off. The medial incision is made as previously described. A full-thickness flap is made using a holding suture to elevate the flap off the undersurface of the tibial sesamoid. Care must be taken to protect the FHL tendon at this point. If shaving is to be performed, 30% to 50% of the plantar surface is planed using a saw while rongeuring or rasping is used to recontour the remaining bone. For grafting, if the tendinous expanse surrounding the sesamoids is intact, then displacement of the repair is unlikely, there-fore no internal fixation is required.[2,5]

The dorsolateral approach is used for fibular sesamoid surgery such as repair of a fibular sesamoid fracture and curettage or grafting of a nonunion. Fibular sesamoid excision can also be achieved using this technique; however, it is more easily per-formed from a plantar incision. A standard 3-cm incision is made in the first interme-tatarsal space dorsally. Dissection is similar to that of a lateral intermetatarsal space release used in bunion surgery. The first structure encountered is the deep transverse intermetatarsal ligament (DTIL). After transecting the DTIL, care is taken to avoid damaging the common digital nerve. The adductor hallucis tendon is removed from the proximal phalanx, lateral aspect of the first MPJ capsule, and lateral fibular sesamoid. This tendon is tagged and retracted and later will be re-approximated for repair. Next, a lateral capsulotomy is performed allowing access to the sesamoid apparatus. The intersesamoidal ligament is then identified and incised to liberate the medial aspect of the fibular sesamoid. Great care is taken to avoid damage to the FHL tendon. Once the fibular sesamoid is removed the metatarsal head and phalangeal base are inspected for cartilaginous defects. Associated defects should be drilled or otherwise repaired as necessary. After completing the procedure, the adductor tendon is reattached to the lateral capsule and a layered closure is per-formed per surgeon's preference.[2,5]

The fourth incisional technique is the plantar approach. To avoid the development of a painful plantar scar, the incision is placed beneath the first intermetatarsal space. A curvilinear incision is made extending from the medial portion near the second digit back to the proximal extent of the metatarsal fat pad. After the incision, the lateral plantar digital nerve of the hallux should be identified and protected either just lateral to the sesamoid or over it. The metatarsal fat pad is retracted medially with the nerve and the fibular sesamoid is then sharply excised from the lateral MTPJ capsule and tendinous attachments of the adductor hallucis and the FHB tendon. Once the sesa-moid has been excised, a layered closure is performed as per the surgeon's prefer-ence. However, the plantar capsular defect should be closed with 2-0 absorbable suture.[2,5]

OSTEOARTHRITIS

Osteoarthritis of the sesamoid apparatus may be secondary to trauma, chondromala-cia, chronic sesamoiditis, hallux rigidus, gout, or rheumatoid arthropathy, among other causes.[5] A common predisposing condition is hallux valgus deformity. As the deformity progresses, the sesamoids become subluxed from the metatarsal and an incongruity occurs within the sesamoid-metatarsal joint. As a result, increased wear on the articular cartilage of the sesamoids and crista evolve and the progression of mechanically induced inflammation leads to degenerative changes which may become symptomatic over time.[2]

INFECTION

Infection involving the sesamoid complex in healthy patients is rare and often results from direct contiguous seeding from adjacent ulcerations in diabetics with peripheral neuropathy (**Fig. 4**). Acute hematogenous spread is possible and primarily occurs in children and young adults from the ages of 9 to 19 years.[2] Treatment of infection includes removal of all infected or potentially infected bone, which can include portions of the metatarsal head or proximal phalanx followed by copious amounts of irrigation and antibiotic therapy is administered based upon the clinical scenario and most often with recommendations from the department of infectious diseases. It is recommended that the surgeon attempts to preserve muscular attachments to prevent a cock-up deformity. When osseous repair is required a staged procedure is planned and the use of internal fixation is delayed until the osteomyelitis is excised or cured. Once the infection is cleared, the hallux can be pinned in plantar flexion for 3 to 4 weeks. A cock-up deformity predisposes the patient to future ulcerations and infections.[5]

INTRACTABLE PLANTAR KERATOSIS

There are numerous causes for intractable plantar keratosis (IPK) of the plantar skin in the region of the sesamoid complex. These lesions may form secondary to structural abnormality of the foot, which includes osteophytosis of the sesamoid complex, dysfunction of the MPJ, a plantar flexed metatarsal, uncompensated forefoot valgus, dorsiflexed second metatarsal, or ankle equinus, among other biomechanical influences (**Fig. 6**). A more diffuse callus can suggest a slightly larger sesamoid or a muscle

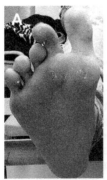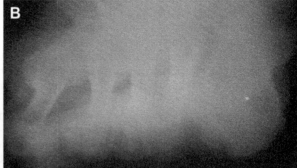

Fig. 6. (*A*) Note the porokeratosis subfibular sesamoid left and sub 2 right associated with gastrocsoleal equinus and brachymetatarsia 3 to 5 bilateral. This 16-year old girl has suffered the ill effects of long-term steroid use in treating dermatomyositis since the age of 5 years. The degree of ankle equinus after progressive tendon contracture contributes to forefoot imbalance and overload, which is her chief complaint. Note the well-circumscribed fat pads inferior to the metatarsal heads. (*B*) The forefoot axial view gives optimal appreciation of the deviation of the sub 1 sesamoid apparatus and the lesser MPJ sesamoids sub 2 and 4 that contribute to the lesion pattern in the left foot seen in (*A*).

imbalance involving the peroneus longus and tibialis anterior or tibialis posterior tendons.[5] Iatrogenic IPKs can result from plantar flexory osteotomies of the first metatarsal, dorsiflexory or shortening osteotomies of the second metatarsal, excision of a singular sesamoid, and a prior shaving procedure on the neighboring sesamoid.[4] While these painful keratoses most often occur in active individuals. These discrete lesions can occur in the athlete and nonathlete alike. When present in the face of diabetic peripheral neuropathy these discrete pressure points can result in ulceration, infection and even direct extension of osteomyelitis into the metatarsal head as seen in **Fig. 4**. Associated soft tissue disorders can be related to IPKs, including a painful bursal sac plantar to the tibial sesamoid (see **Fig. 5**).[2]

Conservative treatment in this case may be as simple as periodic paring and accommodative insoles. For lesions failing routine debridement, surgical treatment may be warranted and can include shaving the plantar surface of the sesamoid or complete excision. Shaving should be avoided when there is a plantar flexed first metatarsal deformity, and excision is contraindicated when the plantar flexed metatarsal is nontranslatable or when the metatarsal rests at a level equal to or above the adjacent metatarsal due to the likelihood of recurrence.[2]

NERVE IMPINGEMENT

The medial or lateral plantar digital nerve can become inflamed for a variety of reasons. The medial plantar digital nerve coursing near the tibial sesamoid becomes irritated because of concomitant hallux valgus deformities as well as overpronation. The lateral plantar digital nerve can be impinged by the fibular sesamoid, but may also produce symptoms of neuritis when the fibular sesamoid is enlarged, displaced, or inflamed itself. Symptoms for nerve impingement include radiating burning pain or numbness distally. Percussion along the route of these nerves with reproduction of the pain can be a telling sign of sesamoid-related nerve impingement.[2,5] A well placed diagnostic block using a short acting local anesthetic agent can help discriminate musculoskeletal causes from nerve irritation.

Treatment of this disorder can be friction-reducing moleskin padding, a wider toe-box to prevent irritation, ultrasound therapy, and deep manual massage. When recalcitrant pain becomes evident, surgical intervention may be warranted. This intervention can include excision of the offending sesamoid with or without external neurolysis and release of the fascial capsular restraints to decompress the region.[5]

SESAMOID FRACTURE

Fractures of the sesamoid can be either acute or stress related, with each displaying different symptoms and imaging characteristics. Regarding sesamoid fracture, the tibial sesamoid is more likely to be affected. Acute fractures of the sesamoids occur because of excessive cyclic weight-bearing loads or direct trauma. They typically present with a sudden onset of plantar pain after a traumatic episode or with repetitive activities. Radiographs may reveal acute fractures as transverse clefts. Each fragment can be varied in size and amount of displacement. Bony calluses can be seen within 2 to 3 weeks, and bone scintigraphy may become positive within 24 hours.[1]

Stress fractures have a slightly different presentation. Onset is generally more gradual and presents after periods of repetitive activity. Radiographic evidence of sesamoidal injury, if it ever manifests, may not be detected for several months. When necessary, CT or MRI can confirm the diagnosis. Stress reactions within the sesamoids share similarities to other stress fractures in bone, but lack the eventual callus formation or obvious cortical disruption. These conditions are nonetheless treated as a stress fracture regarding treatment modalities.[1]

Differentiating the acute fracture from bipartite or multipartitite sesamoids, nonunions and malunions can prove challenging. Bipartite sesamoids generally have smooth-contoured edges as opposed to the irregular trabecular patterns seen in fractures, and a sesamoid can be split into 2, 3, or 4 parts with injury (**Fig. 2**A). It is important to have a high index of suspicion for sesamoid injury or fracture and radiographic comparison with the contra lateral limb is helpful. When the radiographic criteria fit into one of the following categories, the diagnosis of sesamoid fracture is confirmed: (1) an irregular and unequal separation of the affected sesamoid with contours being serrate, (2) evidence of bony callus or attempted healing on serial radiographs, (3) absence of similar radiographic findings in plain films of the contra lateral limb, and (4) surgical treatment with evidence of fracture.[2]

Complications related to both stress fracture and acute fracture include nonunion, malunions, and AVN. A sesamoid is considered a nonunion at an arbitrary time of 6 months, although a more appropriate definition might include a paucity of healing as shown in serial plain films or in ancillary imaging such as CT, NMI, or MRI. Delayed unions or nonunions are more likely to present when the diagnosis of sesamoid disorders has been delayed or missed altogether. The reasons for a missed or delayed diagnosis can include negative radiographs, misinterpreting the pain as FHL tendinitis or 1st MTPJ capsulitis, and the presence of significant concomitant fore foot injury that confounds its presence or simply a patient's own benign neglect. Conservative treatment for sesamoid nonunions is the same as that used for a stress. This treatment includes decreased activity, relative rest via soft cast immobilization and walking boot and often periods of complete immobilization. Surgical intervention, which has been shown by numerous investigators to provide better relief of pain compared with conservative treatment, may consist of excision of the sesamoid, partial excision of the affected sesamoidal pole, and bone grafting.[1] Biedert and Hinterman[6] reported on 5 athletes treated with excision of only the proximal pole of the tibial sesamoid. All 5 athletes returned to activity within 6 months. Anderson and McBryde[10] described using medial eminence autogenous graft for placement in nonunions, and 19 of 21 patients achieved a union and returned to activity. These enhanced and meticulous techniques should not be considered elementary are reserved for the well seasoned foot surgeon.

OSTEOCHONDRITIS AND AVASCULAR NECROSIS (AVN)

This disorder occurs infrequently and is secondary to osseous cell death related to vascular compromise from a varty of conditions. Systemic diseases and medications can be responsible for AVN, but most commonly the culprit is trauma. In the event of trauma (iatrogenic or accidental direct trauma), vascular disruption occurs.[1] Differentiating fracture from avascular necrosis is an important distinction because they can have vastly different long-term outcomes; AVN having the higher incidence of morbidity and dysfunction.

There seems to be a correlation between stress fractures and AVN of the sesamoids. A logical hypothesis is that acute trauma may result in localized disruption to a portion of the vascular supply at the fracture site. The increased marrow edema that results from trauma, prolonged or repetitive weight bearing may lead to widespread ischemia and bone necrosis. Fracture and bony collapse are common sequelae of AVN. AVN of a sesamoid can precipitate a stress fracture, and this explains why they can be recalcitrant to conservative therapy.[1]

The diagnosis of AVN can be aided by radiographs; however, these changes can take up to 6 months following the initial onset of symptoms.[3] Jahss[11] reports radiographic evidence of AVN including early fragmentation, irregularity, and cyst formation. These changes are followed by sclerosis, collapse, flattening, and enlargement of the bone (**Fig. 1**).[11] However, the size of the sesamoids can sometimes make these characteristics difficult to distinguish. To obtain a more accurate diagnosis, a bone scan can be helpful. In the event of an insidious ischemic condition[15] a bone scan reveals a region of decreased isotope uptake, whereas in acute ischemia the surrounding tissues become hyperemic and produce an area of increased uptake. In severe osteonecrosis, the sesamoids do not take up the isotope and a cold spot, or a region of photopenia, becomes evident until revascularization occurs.[2] When MRI is used for this pathology a T1-weighted image with a normal marrow space has been shown to rule out AVN.[1]

THE ROLE OF SESAMOIDS IN HALLUX LIMITUS

Hallux limitus can be debilitating to the patient as it interferes with normal activity and disrupts gait. Generally, it is described as a reduced or absent range of motion usually accompanied by dorsal spurring. Accompanying synovitis or an inflamed bursa may also be present. As mentioned previously, there are numerous and varying causes of hallux limitus or osteoarthritis of the first MPJ. Significant limitation of the 1st MTPJ can result as a consequence of 1st metatarsal elevatus due to trauma or iatrogenic cause. Biomechanical and structural abnormality are culprits for hallux limitus specifically a dorsiflexed first ray, hypermobile first ray, hallux abductovalgus deformity, coalitions within the foot and ankle, a long first metatarsal, and other deformities, have also be associated with the condition. In general the cause of hallux limitus and hallux rigidus is often multifactorial.

The first MPJ is a ball-and-socket joint capable of triplanar motion. In the sagittal plane, the first metatarsal must be capable of plantar flexing and sliding proximally relative to the proximal phalanx. This proximal shift allows the transverse axis to translate dorsally and proximally, which in turn lets the proximal phalanx articulate with the dorsal head of the metatarsal. It is this shift in the transverse axis that allows the first MPJ to increase the range of dorsiflexion during propulsion as opposed to that seen in static stance. Therefore, it is proposed that anything limiting the first metatarsal from plantar flexing or shifting proximally would limit the shift of the transverse axis and ultimately decrease dorsiflexion at that joint.[12]

Durrant and Siepert[12] believe that, to effectively restrict dorsiflexion at the first MPJ, the plantar structures must cross the transverse axis of motion, lie below the transfer axis of motion, attach to the distal hinge or proximal phalanx, exert a force that is parallel to the longitudinal axis of the first metatarsal, and be present on both sides of the longitudinal axis of the first ray. They believe that the sesamoids, FHB, joint capsule, and medial plantar fascial band meet this criterion.[12]

Because of the encasement of the sesamoids in the FHB tendons, it is necessary to understand how each can restrict first MPJ range of motion. The origin of the FHB is on the lateral cuneiform and cuboid and crosses the transverse axis to insert on the proximal phalanx and in doing so it meets all of the criteria described by Durrant and Siepert.[12] The FHB is a stance phase muscle that acts from midstance through the end of propulsion by stabilizing the proximal phalanx against the metatarsal head and ground. Therefore, its anatomic position can limit dorsiflexion if the muscle causes excessive tension against the inferior surface of the metatarsal. This tension happens when the muscle is short compared with the length of the first metatarsal or in the presence of sesamoids. If there is excessive plantar tension, then there is increased stress placed on the dorsal head of the metatarsal by the base of the proximal phalanx, a retrograde force, which, in time, causes bone reactive changes and dorsal spurring.[12] Mann[13] commented that intrinsic muscles of the foot have to work harder in a pronated foot type during midstance and propulsion, which increases plantar tension. This explains why hallux limitus is commonly associated with a pronated foot type.

The sesamoids have an intricate connection with the FHB tendons because they enhance the pulley action of the tendon and subsequently the muscle's function. The sesamoid position relative to the first MPJ has not been fully evaluated.[12] According to Root and colleagues,[14] biomechanically the sesamoids assume a more distal position as the first ray plantar flexes and moves posteriorly. The pulley system becomes activated at heel-off, and the first metatarsal head glides proximally on the sesamoid apparatus. In order for this pulley system to operate properly, the sesamoids must be located exactly at the joint where the FHB tendons turn to attach to the proximal phalanx.[12,14] Problems arise when the sesamoid apparatus is proximally located and fixed as can be seen in later stages of hallux rigidus. This condition has a domino effect on the first MPJ, with a decrease in the plantar flexion and motion of the first metatarsal, which in turn prevents the transverse axis of the 1st MTPJ from moving dorsally and proximally. This limitation of motion prompts dorsal joint abutment and excessive jamming of the proximal phalanx on the metatarsal head.[12] Camasta[15] correlates dysfunction of the 1st MTPJ with a retraction or spasm of the FHB resulting in a proximal position of the sesamoid apparatus; a secondary response to painful arthroses. Initial inferior jamming on the sesamoid apparatus can result in erosive changes along the sesamoid grooves that can be visualized at the time of surgery.[15]

Generally, anything that limits first metatarsal plantar flexion eventually leads to hallux limitus. As mentioned previously, proximally displaced sesamoids play a role. However, other sesamoid abnormalities may contribute as well. Elongation of the sesamoids, as occurs due to traction osteophytosis, can prevent plantar flexion of the metatarsal. Bipartite sesamoids, whether congenital or resulting from fracture, are generally longer in the transverse plane of the foot. This morphology results from the excessive pressures of first metatarsal plantar flexion at the time of toe-off. A deep or hypertrophic sesamoid, whether congenital or secondary to osteoarthritis, limits the first metatarsal plantar flexion and sets off the cascade of hallux limitus development.[12,16]

Most sesmoid pathologies involve chronic inflammation and so there is over lap in these syndromes and so it is important to assess the radiographs and each individual clinical scenario carefully. Sesamoids may contain several characteristics that lead to hallux limitus or hallux rigidus. The natural location of the sesamoid apparatus is predictable as it is deeply invested in its' fibrocapsular environment and this was proven reported by Judge and colleagues[17] as it related to hallux abducto valgus surgery. The dogma that existed over decades of HAV surgery perpetuated the notion that the sesamoids were released of adhesions and were relocated as a result of HAV surgery. After measuring the position of the tibial sesamoid as it related to the 2nd metatarsal it was statistically established that the sesamoid apparatus in fact does not move and is fixed within its soft tissue environment even as a result of HAV surgery. Consequently it was proven that the translocation of the first metatarsal over the sesamoids is what gives the appearance of sesamoid migration in postoperative films in HAV surgery.

In 1949, Harris and Beath[18] believed the normal distance of the sesamoids from the 1st MTPJ was 12.5 mm to 16.5 mm. Without citing specific values, Yoshioka and colleagues[19] stated that the fibular sesamoid was further from the distal portion of the first metatarsal. Prieskorn and colleagues[20] and Hetherington and colleagues[21] both found mean distances to be shorter than those given by Harris and Beath.[18] Prieskorn and colleagues[20] found a mean distance of 4.9 mm of the tibial sesamoid and 7.6 mm of the fibular sesamoid, whereas Hetherington and colleagues[21] found a mean distance of the tibial sesamoid to be 5.7 mm. Munuera and colleagues[22] found values similar to those of Hetherington and colleagues[21] and Prieskorn and colleagues[20] and their data agree with the proposal by Yoshioka and colleagues[19]that the tibial sesamoid is located closer to the joint.[16] Roukis and colleagues[23] studied feet diagnosed with hallux rigidus and examined the distance of the sesamoids from the joint. They concluded that there was slight proximal migration of the sesamoids when comparing their data with the normal mean values of Hetherington and colleagues[21] and Prieskorn and colleagues.[20] In a study by Munuera and colleagues[22] that examined 183 radiographs, there was no significance found in the distance of the sesamoids from the joint in feet with hallux limitus compared with normal feet. However, there was significance in the length of the sesamoid bones themselves in hallux limitus. No other prior studies had examined sesamoid size in patients with normal and hallux limitus feet.[16,22] Studies had been performed that examined normal values. Oloff and Schulhofer[1] found the tibial sesamoid to be larger and the fibular sesamoid to be rounder. Yoshioka and colleagues[19] agreed and found the tibial sesamoid in normal feet to be 10.6 mm, whereas the fibular sesamoid was 10.1 mm. Aper and colleagues[24,25] reported a normal fibular sesamoid to be 13.61 mm.

SURGERY IN THE HALLUX LIMITUS FOOT IN RELATION TO SESAMOID CAUSES

Generally, when evaluating a hallux limitus or rigidus deformity for surgery, the surgeon considers several procedures, usually without taking the sesamoid characteristics into account. Procedures commonly used include simple cheilectomies, first MTPJ arthrodeses, plantar flexory and shortening distal osteotomies, and joint replacement procedures. To have a successful outcome, these procedures should meet certain criteria. Distal osteotomies on the first metatarsal should allow for a stable shortening and an ability to adjust increases in the declination angle of the metatarsal. This osteotomy should allow for ample resection of dorsal cartilage of the first metatarsal head. Also, the plantar cartilage and sesamoidal grooves should be preserved.[12,16]

Root and colleagues[14] believed that any osteotomy that shortens the first metatarsal should also plantar flex, which addresses the more proximal location of the sesamoids and the plantar jamming resultant from the virtual lengthening of the plantar intrinsics as the metatarsal is shortened. The combination of these maneuvers allows the sesamoids to translate distally as the 1st MTPJ is put through stance and the propulsive phase of gait. This action concurrently relieves the proximal axial pressure of the proximal phalanx on the metatarsal head. The Youngswick osteotomy has been shown to shorten the metatarsal and plantarflex the metatarsal head and can be used in a metatarsal that is normal length with no hypermobility or dorsiflexion, but with elongated sesamoids.[12,26] The original Watermann osteotomy, wedge resection of the dorsal metatarsal head rotating the plantar cartilage into the MTPJ, succeeded in shortening the first metatarsal without plantar flexing and seems to be effective when the sesamoids are hypertrophic instead of proximally translocated. Osteotomies can also be performed proximally at the base or shaft and, when needed, a Lapidus procedure can be used to shorten and plantar flex the metatarsal while maintaining range of motion of the first MTPJ.[12,16]

In selecting the cheilectomy procedure or one of its modifications sesamoid excision may be performed as an adjunctive procedure for grades I & II hallux limitus and the risks associated with that maneuver are well understood. Tagoe and colleagues[27] performed a retrospective study on 33 patients with total sesamoidectomy for grade I or II hallux limitus with a normal or even a short first metatarsal. This study reported no complications and favorable subjective outcomes between 2 and 4 years of follow-up. Aper and colleagues[25] examined the effect of sesamoid resection on the effective moment arm of the FHB and FHL tendons in cadaveric studies. For the FHB tendon, a significant decrease in the moment arm occurred only when both sesamoids were removed. A significant decrease in the moment arm of the FHL tendon was noted after removal of each sesamoid individually and with total sesamoidectomies. However, no significant change was noted when hemiresections were performed, indicating that partial sesamoidectomy can be performed without significant compromise in the strength of the FHL tendon.[24]

Controversy still remains concerning the role of the sesamoids in hallux limitus and how these small ossicles should be addressed surgically. A limited amount of evidenced-based literature is available on the matter and even that generally has a low level of evidence. As with most questions regarding sesamoid pathology further evidenced based medicine is required to reconcile controversy in this matter.

ACKNOWLEDGMENTS

Acknowledgment and heartfelt appreciation is extended to the medical library and audiovisual staff members of St Vincent Mercy Hospital Toledo, OH, for assistance in procuring articles and reproducing illustrations.

REFERENCES

1. Oloff L, Schulhofer D. Sesamoid complex disorders. Clin Podiatr Med Surg 1996; 13(3):497–513.
2. Dedmond B, Cory JW, McBryde A Jr. The hallucal sesamoid complex. J Am Acad Orthop Surg 2006;14:745–53.
3. Sanders T, Rathur S. Imaging of painful conditions of the hallucal sesamoid complex and plantar capsular structures of the first metatarsophalangeal joint. Radiol Clin North Am 2008;46:1079–92.
4. Cohen B. Hallux sesamoid disorders. Foot Ankle Clin N Am 2009;14:91–104.
5. Richardson E. Hallucal sesamoid pain: causes and surgical treatment. J Am Acad Orthop Surg 1999;7:270–8.
6. Biedert R, Hintermann B. Stress fractures of the medial great toe sesamoids in athletes. Foot Ankle Int 2003;24(2):137–41.
7. Weil L, Hill M. Bipartite tibial sesamoid and hallux abductovalgus deformity: a previously unreported correlation. J Foot Surg 1992;31(2):104–11.
8. Speed K. Injuries of the great toe sesamoids. Ann Surg 1914;60(4):478–80.
9. Aquino MD, DeVincentis AF, Keating SE. Tibial sesamoid planing procedure: an appraisal of 26 feet. J Foot Surg 1984;23(3):226–30.
10. Anderson RB, McBryde AM. Autogenous bone grafting hallux sesamoid nonunions. Foot Ankle Int 1997;18(5):293–6.
11. Jahss MH. The sesamoids of the hallux. Clin Orthop Relat Res 1981;157:88–97.
12. Durrant M, Siepert K. Role of soft tissue structures as an etiology of hallux limitus. J Am Podiatr Med Assoc 1993;83(4):173–80.
13. Mann R, editor. Surgery of the foot. St Louis (MO): CV Mosby; 1986. p. 10.

14. Root ML, Orien WP, Weed JH, et al. Normal and abnormal function of the foot, clinical biomechanics, vol. II. Los Angeles (CA): Clinical Biomechanics; 1977.
15. Camasta C. Hallux limitus and hallux rigidus: clinical examination, radiographic findings, and natural history. Clin Podiatr Med Surg 1996;13(3):423–48.
16. Zammit G, Menz HB, Munteanu SE. Structural factors associated with hallux limitus/rigidus: a systematic review of case controlled studies. J Orthop Sports Phys Ther 2009;39(10):733–42.
17. Judge MS, LaPointe S, Yu GV, et al. Hallux valgus surgery and the sesamoid apparatus; a critical statistical analysis. William J. Stickle Gold Award. J Am Podiatr Med Assoc 1999;89(11/12).
18. Harris RI, Beath T. The short first metatarsal; its incidence and clinical significance. J Bone Joint Surg Am 1949;31(3):553–65.
19. Yoshioka Y, Siu DW, Cooke TD, et al. Geometry of the first metatarsophalangeal joint. J Orthop Res 1998;6:878.
20. Prieskorn D, Graves SC, Smith RA. Morphometric analysis of the plantar plate apparatus of the first metatarsophalangeal joint. Foot Ankle 1993;14(4):204–7.
21. Hetherington V, Carnett J, Patterson BA. Motion of the first metatarsophalangeal joint. J Foot Surg 1989;28(1):13–9.
22. Munuera P, Dominguez G, Lafuente G. Length of the sesamoids and their distance from the metatarsophalangeal joint space in feet with incipient hallux limitus. J Am Podiatr Med Assoc 2008;98(2):123–9.
23. Roukis T, Jacobs PM, Dawson DM, et al. A prospective comparison of clinical, radiographic, and intraoperative features of hallux rigidus. J Foot Ankle Surg 2002;41(2):76–95.
24. Aper R, Saltzman CL, Brown TD. The effect of hallux sesamoid excision on the flexor hallucis longus moment arm. Clin Orthop Relat Res 1996;325:209–17.
25. Aper R, Saltzman CL, Brown TD, et al. The effect of hallux sesamoid resection on the effective moment of the flexor hallucis brevis. Foot Ankle Int 1994;15:462–9.
26. Youngswick FD. Modifications of the Austin bunionectomy for treatment of metatarsus primus elevatus associated with hallux limitus. J Foot Surg 1982;21(2):114–6.
27. Tagoe M, Brown HA, Rees SM. Total sesamoidectomy for painful hallux rigidus: a medium-term outcome study. Foot Ankle Int 2009;30(7):640–6.

Modern Techniques in Hallux Abducto Valgus Surgery

Bradly W. Bussewitz, DPM, AACFAS[a], Tim Levar, DPM[b],
Christopher F. Hyer, DPM[a],*

KEYWORDS

- Lapidus • Locked plate • Opening wedge plate
- TightRope • Bunion • Akin • Staple

OPENING BASE WEDGE

The opening base wedge (OBW) osteotomy for correction of hallux abducto valgus (HAV) and hallux primus varus (HPV) was introduced by Trethowan in 1923.[1] His technique described a hinged osteotomy with interposition of a wedge-shaped graft. He did not recommend fixation. This lack of fixation and perhaps the lack of quality fixation over the years provided the OBW few supporters throughout history. The osteotomy is vulnerable to hinge fracture and subsequent elevation of the capital arm, as well as delayed union or nonunion. Jamming of the first metatarsal phalangeal joint is also a recognized concern. Other, more reliable procedures were preferred for moderate to severe HAV correction. The scarf, crescentic, closing base wedge, and Lapidus are more frequently used because they are more stable and thus predictable.

Medical device innovation has brought the OBW into focus for HAV surgery. The procedure-specific OBW plate is the focus of this section. To effectively open the medial base of the wedge on the first metatarsal, the lateral hinge has to be made sufficiently thin; if the hinge is too thick, it will likely fracture as the wedge is pried opened (**Fig. 1**). The ability of the plate to offload the ground reactive forces, caused by weight bearing, on the intact hinge allows the bone to incorporate into the gap, with diminished risk of fracture or disruption during the postoperative course. An "efficient" osteotomy should be performed at 90° to the medial border of the metatarsal; at this angle, screw fixation is difficult. Landing a screw across a narrow bone at such an acute angle offers less than ideal fixation strength and compression according to arbeitsgemeinschaft osteosynthesefragen (AO) principles.

Financial disclosure: Dr Christopher Hyer is a consultant for Wright Medical.
[a] Orthopedic Foot and Ankle Center, 300 Polaris Parkway Suite 2000, Westerville, OH 43082, USA
[b] Cleveland Clinic Foundation, c/o GME - NA23 - Podiatry, 9500 Euclid Avenue, Cleveland, OH 44195, USA
* Corresponding author.
E-mail address: ofacresearch@orthofootankle.com

Clin Podiatr Med Surg 28 (2011) 287–303
doi:10.1016/j.cpm.2011.03.005
0891-8422/11/$ – see front matter © 2011 Elsevier Inc. All rights reserved.
podiatric.theclinics.com

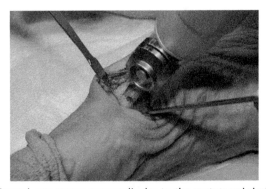

Fig. 1. Medial to lateral osteotomy, perpendicular to the metatarsal shaft.

Recent literature has supported the use of a low-profile plate and screw system (Arthrex Inc, Naples, FL, USA) designed specifically for a basilar opening wedge procedure (**Fig. 2**).[2–6] The plate has many desirable features. The first is its low profile design. The medial cortex of the first metatarsal has minimal soft tissue buffering from local nerves and the skin. Any prominence in this area often leads to painful hardware and neurologic symptoms. The design of the plate to adhere closely to the bone and of the screws to seat down into the plate minimizes protrusion risks. The plate also features a solid wedge that is offset from the wall of the plate. The wedge allows seating of the plate into a reproducible location and holds the osteotomy at a predictable gap distance.

In 2009 several articles related to the Arthrex plate were published, whose authors' excitement was palpable. Cooper and colleagues,[7] Wukich and colleagues,[8] and Hardy and Grove[2] all described the OBW technique and described plate features. The technique is technical but reproducible. Of critical importance is maintaining a lateral cortical hinge without fracture as well as avoidance of first met base medial cuneiform joint violation with the osteotomy and the screws. Techniques vary regarding the orientation of the cut; some choose to remain perpendicular to the

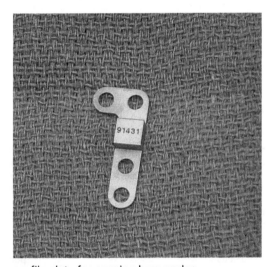

Fig. 2. Arthrex low-profile plate for opening base wedge.

ground whereas others prefer to remain perpendicular to the first metatarsal shaft, and yet others split the difference. Ideally the cut should be performed with a purpose based on the biomechanical specifics of the particular case (**Fig. 3**).

A radiographic evaluation of 29 patients with 31 OBW procedures treated with the plate was retrospectively analyzed. The 3.5-mm, 4.0-mm, and 5.0-mm wedge plates had a mean first intermetatarsal angle correction of 8°, 9°, and 14.9°, respectively. The investigators described the procedure as "highly effective for correcting moderate to severe intermetatarsal (IM) deformities."[3] Wukich and colleagues[4] reviewed 18 OBW procedures using the Arthrex plate, 3 years after writing the technique guide. The investigators found the IM angle improved by a mean of 9°, the hallux valgus angle improved by 13.5°, and the metatarsal protrusion distance increased by 2.6 mm. The preoperative and postoperative Seiberg index did not show a statistical significance. Sixteen of 18 (89%) patients reported satisfaction with the procedure. A similar study examined 46 patients with 64 procedures using the Arthrex plate. The hallux abductus angle (HAA) and IM angle improved an average of 14.7° and 6.4°, respectively. Complications included 5 hallux varus; one was symptomatic and there was one nonunion, which required bone grafting. American Orthopaedic Foot and Ankle Society (AOFAS) scoring improved from 51.3 to 86.8.[5]

Shurnas and colleagues[6] retrospectively examined 78 patients, including 84 OBW procedures with the Arthrex plate. IM improvement averaged 9.9°, HAA decreased by 20°. Average time to radiographic union was 5.9 weeks. There were one nonunion, one delayed union, 4 hallux varus, and 3 recurrences, with no plate failures. Ninety percent of the patients reported good to excellent results. The patients were allowed to immediately bear weight postoperatively.

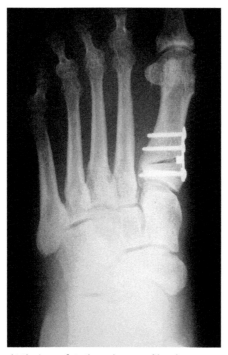

Fig. 3. Anteroposterior (AP) view of Arthrex low-profile plate postoperatively.

The significance of early weight bearing has numerous benefits. Patients can return to activities faster, avoid disuse atrophy, and reduce the risk of deep vein thrombosis by decreasing stasis and increasing lower extremity muscle milking. Incorporating locking-plate technology with a wedged plate can arguably strengthen the construct, allowing better results, particularly with early weight-bearing goals.

The Darco Base Opening Wedge (BOW) Plate (Wright Medical Technology, Inc, Arlington, TN, USA) is analogous to the Arthrex plate. The plate is similarly titanium with a wedge of variable sizes. The theoretical improvement of the BOW plate is the locking capability of the plate (**Fig. 4**). The 2.7-mm screws can be locked as a fixed angle construct or nonlocked at variable degrees, depending on the specific needs of the patient. Also, using the drill guides as levers, the plate can be easily contoured to the bone to perfectly match the medial contour of the first metatarsal base. The titanium alloy is adequately strong yet malleable enough to allow for appropriate contouring. The locking ability increases the strength of the construct. If the patient were to bear too much weight in the initial postoperative course, the cortical hinge might fracture and the metatarsal might elevate or create a delay in healing (**Fig. 5**). The lateral hinge may also be iatrogenically broken during the procedure, and the added strength provided by the fixed-angle construct may prove valuable.

Smith and colleagues[9] examined 49 osteotomies on 47 patients, 32 of whom were fitted with the BOW plate. These investigators found a 1- to 2-IM correction of 7°, and noted 4 (8%) delayed union and nonunion, all of which occurred in the nonlocking plate group. None of the locking plate groups developed a delay in healing (**Fig. 6**). In summary, they recommended the use of the locking system. The trend in foot and ankle surgery is to incorporate locking-plate technology into patients or surgeries that are "at risk." The OBW is an inherently unstable osteotomy in a critical weight-bearing location. A strong argument can be made for a fixed-angle construct to protect this osteotomy until boney consolidation.

Use of bone graft to backfill the opening wedge site can be performed with the OBW. The medial eminence from the distal Silver bunionectomy can be used, and a cancellous allograft or a demineralized bone matrix has also been documented. The cost versus biologic benefit needs to be considered when using additional products, however. It seems logical to backfill with graft particularly in the at-risk patients, as well as those with an extreme wedge size and a resultant large bone deficit at the wedge site. Shurnas and colleagues[6] supports usage of the medial eminence, Saragas[5] used the medial eminence or harvested autogenous cancellous bone from

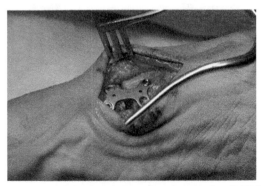

Fig. 4. Intraoperative picture of the Darco Base Opening Wedge (BOW) plate.

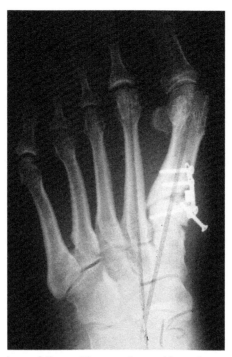

Fig. 5. AP view of hardware failure with nonunion and loss of correction with nonlocking plate and screws.

the distal tibia, and Hardy and Grove[2] described using the medial eminence and allo-graft bone chips to fill the void, as did Cooper and colleagues.[7]

OBW-specific plates have rejuvenated the foot and ankle community regarding basilar HAV procedures. Unlike the first metatarsal cuneiform fusion, the OBW is joint sparing and offers a similarly powerful corrective ability. Literature on surgical technique is available to offer the OBW novice an inside look at technical pearls. Those currently using the OBW and its associated plates are producing articles to allow others to realize the successes and failures they are experiencing. Newer fixation technologies will continue to surface to augment the currently available products. The future of the OBW appears bright.

LOCKED-PLATE LAPIDUS

Paul Lapidus popularized a first tarsometatarsal arthrodesis procedure, detailing "his" methods in a 1934 article.[10] His initial procedure used cat-gut suture to fixate the prepared fusion site. Fixation has changed dramatically over the years. The Lapidus procedure is widely used throughout the world. Whether one is treating hypermobility, joint arthritis, moderate or severe metatarsus primus, or HAV, the Lapidus can be useful. The powerful corrective ability and low rate of deformity recurrence affords the procedure popularity.

The Lapidus is not without its drawbacks. There is a relatively high rate of delayed union or nonunion reports in the literature. It can be technically challenging to reproduce exact correction and, perhaps most frustrating both for the physician and the patient, is the convalescent period that has been tagged to the procedure.

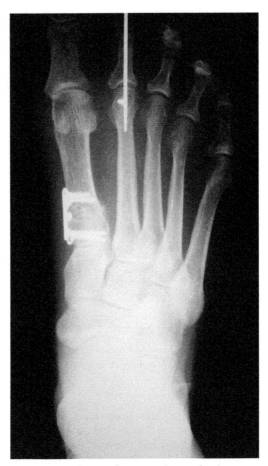

Fig. 6. AP view of locking BOW plate with appropriate reduction.

Unfortunately, at times surgeons choose a less indicated procedure to obviate the long convalescence period. Fortunately, innovative plate and screw designs have decreased the time to weight bearing postoperatively.

Numerous investigators have produced studies and reviews to help guide the explosion in locking-plate opportunities and technologies during recent years. Fixed-angle constructs are taking many shapes and capabilities. Precontouring, bending or malleability potential, eccentric compression capabilities, variable angle lock features, low-profile designs, and even color choices offer the surgeon a great "tackle box" to choose from. The Lapidus procedure has specifically been the focus of studies to determine the benefits locking plates offer, if any, over traditional fixation methods.

Nonunion rates have been reported as high as 12%.[11–15] Many reasons can be blamed for poor fusion rates. The medial cuneiform is relatively small, necessitating smaller hardware and also less than ideal hardware landing. The joint is notorious for inadequate preparation, perhaps due to its depth and tight soft tissue package. Perhaps the most important reason for failure is that the ground reactive forces are focused at the plantar, tension, side of this particular arthrodesis. The vector of force encourages diastasis at the plantar side of the fusion. Attention to joint preparation detail and fixation aimed at neutralizing the extreme plantar forces is the focus for decreasing delayed union, nonunion, and malunion.

The evolution of construct design and technique has brought successes and failures when comparing traditional screw fixation and fixed-angle plating. Cohen and colleagues[16] showed that a dorsomedial locking plate without an additional compression screw was inferior to a crossed-screw construct in metatarsal cuneiform fusions. The investigators focused on the inability of the plate to negate the plantar tension forces and the lack of compression afforded without a compression screw.

In a cadaver study, Gruber and colleagues[17] compared a traditional crossed 4.0 screw construct to a dorsomedial locking plate with adjunct screw compression. The specimens were loaded to failure. There was no difference in load to failure or stiffness. The fact that the plate was placed medial should provide improved strength against tension forces, especially with a compression screw to create friction, and thus stability, at the interface.

Marks and colleagues[18] found that a nonlocking plate fixed to the plantar aspect of the joint had a significantly higher failure point than screw fixation. The major force with weight bearing imparted on a metatarsal cuneiform joint is from the plantar side. It then makes sense that some type of plantar plate or lower medial plate would better oppose these forces, and Marks showed this, even with a nonlocking plate. Unfortunately, because of the dense soft tissue package plantarly, plate placement here is difficult in vivo, especially when trying to insert screws.

Scranton and colleagues[19] performed a cadaveric study comparing a locked dorsal Lapidus plate with compression screw versus conventional 4.0 crossed screws. A higher load to failure and bending moment was noted in the plate group. The plate used in this study was designed specifically for the Lapidus fusion. This construct of a lock plate and compression screw correlates with the promising "real-world" outcomes in the literature.

The clinical outcomes for the lock plate with interfragment screw are encouraging, despite a mixed cadaveric review of fixation strengths. Saxena and colleagues[20] showed in a level II study that there was no difference in postoperative complications between locking plate with screw construct and a crossed lag screw design. The crossed-screw group was allowed to bear weight at the traditional 6 weeks, whereas the plate group was allowed to bear weight at only 4 weeks. To effectively compare fixation, the control crossed-screw group would ideally be allowed to bear weight at 4 weeks as well, but the standard of care for crossed screws remains at 6 to 8 weeks.

Sorensen and colleagues[21] evaluated the results of Lapidus arthrodesis with locked plating and early weight bearing. The average radiographic fusion time was 6.95 weeks, time to weight bearing was 2 weeks, and the investigators saw a 9.52% asymptomatic malunion rate and a 0% rate of delayed union or nonunion. These results support the benefits of a locked-plate construct with compression screw.

The literature jury seems to favor lock plating with interfragment screw compression (**Fig. 7**) over traditional fixation, especially when a shorter convalescence period is considered. Cadaveric studies lack the features of real-life dynamics. The tissue no doubt undergoes changes post mortem, which could alter outcomes. The loading features, no matter how intuitive the study design, do not perfectly imitate actual weight-bearing loads. The plate also allows more bone on bone-healing surface area otherwise obscured by the screw as it traverses the joint, which shields bone formation at the screw site (**Fig. 8**). Possible other, unforeseen, differences may also play a role. Thus the in vivo studies by Sorensen and colleagues[21] and Saxena and colleagues[20] promote the success of early weight bearing and lock-plate fixation over standard screw fixation and longer convalescent periods.

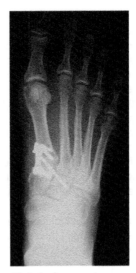

Fig. 7. AP view of locked plate with interfragment screw.

Lock plating is here to stay in foot and ankle surgery. Plate designs and fixation construct differences continue to evolve. The Lapidus HAV procedure has withstood the test of time. As surgeons continue to publish their results, best practices can be established. Allowing an earlier return to weight bearing and normal shoe gear will

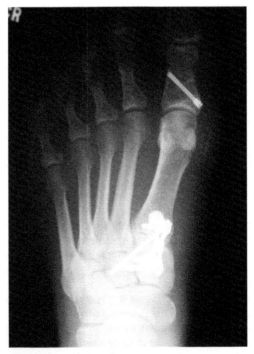

Fig. 8. AP view of locked plate with interfragment screw.

allow surgeons to use this procedure when moderate and severe bunions are present, even when return to activity is of high priority to patients.

TIGHTROPE AND HAV

Recently, the TightRope device (Arthrex Inc, Naples, FL, USA) has been used to recreate anatomic ligaments and tendons in several conditions, including reconstruction of acromioclavicular joint dislocations[22] and ankle syndesmotic disruptions (**Fig. 9**).[23] However, there is no direct anatomic ligamentous attachment from the distal aspect of the first metatarsal to the second metatarsal to "recreate."[24] Placement of an interosseous suture and button device for correction of a hallux valgus deformity creates a structure analogous to a ligament that is not present (**Figs. 10** and **11**).[25] The Mini TightRope is indicated for Lisfranc ligament repair, hallux varus, and hallux valgus repair, and for hallux valgus deformities with congruent joint with an IM angle less than 15°.[26,27] When the FiberWire (Arthrex, Naples, FL, USA) is tightened, the IM angle is reduced to a desired value (<9–11°). The Mini TightRope can be used with a distal osteotomy for larger IM angles or semi-rigid deformities.[27]

The correction of a hallux valgus deformity with the suture button first involves the assessment of the hallux valgus angle, intermetatarsal angle, any interphalangeous deformity, and distal metatarsal articular angle. It is also important to assess for the presence or absence of any arthritic involvement of the first metatarsophalangeal joint and first metatarsocuneiform joint. According to Holmes,[26] the tightrope is contraindicated in the presence of arthrosis or dorsoplantar hypermobility of the first metatarsocuneiform joint, a proximal first metatarsal facet abutting the base of the second metatarsal, arthrosis of the first metatarsophalangeal joint, lateral angulation of the distal metatarsal articular angle, and large congruent deformities. Holmes advocated obtaining a detailed history questioning the presence of rheumatoid arthritis, diabetes, gout, systemic inflammatory arthropathies, or neuromuscular disorders, and the presence of one or more of these disorders should be a relative contraindication to using the Mini TightRope.[26]

In a recent study by Ponnapula and Wittock,[25] a retrospective analysis was performed on 5 female patients with a mild to moderate bunion deformity, defined as a first IM angle between 9° and 15°, whereby an interosseous suture and button device was used to correct a HAV deformity. Three of the patients received the standard technique whereby the interosseous suture was placed through the proximal portion of the second metatarsal neck. In the alternative technique, the interosseous suture was

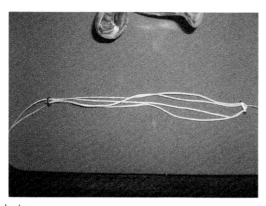

Fig. 9. TightRope device.

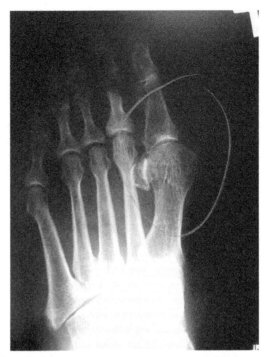

Fig. 10. Preoperative AP view.

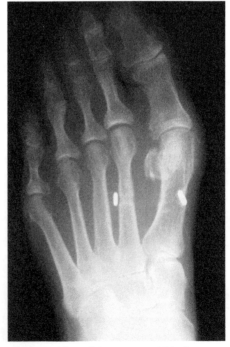

Fig. 11. Postoperative AP view with endobutton at midshaft.

placed in the proximal portion of the diaphysis of the second metatarsal. The median postoperative reduction in the first IM angle was 5° and the median postoperative reduction in the HAA was 17°. Statistically significant reductions in the long-term first intermetatarsal angles and HAAs were also seen.

In a case report by West,[28] the TightRope procedure and hemi-joint implant was used in a 68-year-old well-controlled diabetic female with a history of 2 episodes of deep venous thrombosis occurring after previous surgery with immobilization in a below-the-knee cast. The preoperative intermetatarsal angle was measured at 22.5°, with an HAA of 48°. The immediate postoperative radiographic measurements demonstrated a corrected intermetatarsal angle of 6° and a corrected HAA of 8°, and 9° and 8.5° at 18 months, respectively. The utility of a minimally invasive procedure with a short convalescent period makes the TightRope a valuable tool.

The Mini TightRope was developed to eliminate most of the complications and potential risks associated with other distal and proximal metatarsal osteotomies[27] including delayed union, malunion, nonunion, shortening of the first metatarsal, avascular necrosis, hardware failure, and prolonged protected ambulation. In addition, some have advocated that decreased first metatarsophalangeal joint motion, shortening of the first metatarsal, dorsal displacement of the capital fragment, and transfer metatarsalgia are other complications associated with distal metatarsal osteotomies.[29] This procedure, not unlike other documented procedures, does carry potential risks and complications.

Holmes[26] described fracture of the second metatarsal as a potential complication of the application of the TightRope device in 10% of patients. It was concluded that the development of acute fractures was from increased stress risers of the narrowing of second metatarsal. Late asymptomatic second metatarsal fractures have been reported when the second intermetatarsal ligament was not released.[26] In the previously described analysis of 5 patients undergoing application of an interosseous suture device by Ponnapula and Wittock,[25] all 5 of their patients developed complications. The complications included fracture of the second metatarsal, stress fracture of the fourth metatarsal, a case of hallux varus, and a recurrent case of hallux abductus. The investigators felt that the larger circumference of the metatarsal at a more proximal level may have lessened the stress of the device on the cortex. The study also concluded that less movement occurred with more proximal placement of the device, which led to more favorable outcomes based on the premise that the arc of metatarsal excursion is larger distally than proximally.

In a case report by Kemp and colleagues,[30] a 73-year-old woman underwent an endobutton repair for recurrent hallux valgus. In this case, proximal and distal Mini TightRope implants were used. Five weeks after the procedure, a fracture through the distal drill hole in the second metatarsal was seen, leading to loss of fixation of the TightRope and recurrent hallux valgus, treated with open reduction and internal fixation and removal of the distal device.

Mader and Han[31] reported on bilateral second metatarsal stress fractures after hallux valgus correction with the use of a tension wire and button fixation device. In this case report, a 22-year-old woman underwent bilateral hallux valgus. At postoperative week 20, radiographs revealed bilateral stress fractures at the site of the tunnel in the second metatarsal. In a study that measured the ultimate load to failure of the second metatarsal with drill holes placed proximally and distally, it was found that the proximally placed tunnel failed at a lower ultimate load than did the distally placed tunnel, with fractures occurring through the tunnels.[32]

The Arthrex Mini TightRope device provides an alternative means to reduce and maintain the intermetatarsal angle, while avoiding the complications associated with other conventional first metatarsal osteotomies in the correction of HAV deformities. The tightrope may have merit in the surgical treatment of patients with associated comorbidities whereby conventional first metatarsal osteotomies are not indicated based on the required postoperative course.[28] According to the literature, the suture endobutton does reduce the intermetatarsal and hallux abduction angle in a hallux valgus deformity following correct placement of the device.[25,28,31] However, there have been reports of potential complications with the use of the device, most notably second metatarsal fracture. The initial outcomes are based on small case reports and retrospective analyses of small groups of patients, all with limited postoperative follow-up. Further long-term studies with larger patient populations are needed to assess the efficacy and validity of this modern fixation device for the correction of a hallux valgus deformity.

AKIN AND STAPLE FIXATION

In 1925, Akin described a surgical procedure consisting of resection of the medial eminence of the first metatarsal head as well as a portion of bone from the base of the proximal phalanx.[33] The procedure also included a medial closing wedge osteotomy of the proximal phalanx of the hallux. Since 1925, this osteotomy and its various modifications have been widely used in clinical practice. The Akin has been described as an additional corrective procedure combined with first metatarsal osteotomies including the chevron or Scarf osteotomies.[34,35] It is indicated when an interphalangeal deformity persists after correction of the IM angle, distal metatarsal articular angle, and the hallux valgus angle by other osseous procedures and soft tissue rebalancing.[36] Several methods of fixation have been described over the years. Fixation of the Akin osteotomy historically has included splinting, Kirschner wires, monofilament wire, and screw fixation.[37,38] With modern advances in metal alloy engineering and absorbable materials, several types of bone staples are now being used for the fixation of Akin osteotomies (**Figs. 12** and **13**).

Bone staples have been widely used in foot and ankle surgery. The advantages of fixation with staples include approximation of the bone fragments, dynamic compression, avoidance of pin-tract infections, and less operating time compared with screws.[39] The use of power-driven staples was associated with a 33% decrease in operating time for internal fixation of ankle fractures as compared with pin and screw fixation.[40]

Compression staples are an alternative form of internal fixation that provides either static or dynamic compression to two surfaces. The two main designs of compression staples available are mechanical and shape memory. The designs differ in their mode of activation. Mechanical compression staples rely on mechanical manipulation of the staple to achieve compression, whereas shape memory staples reach their intended shape by reaching a temperature higher than its storage temperature.[41]

Many types of bone staples are available. The current goal of staple manufacturers is to improve the strength, stability, and ease of use by implant designs and by altering metal composition. Nitinol is an acronym that stands for nickel (Ni), titanium (Ti), and Naval Ordinance Laboratory (NOL), where the alloy was discovered in the 1960s. Nitinol is a metal alloy with "shape memory" controlled by temperature.[42]

Nitinol is being used in several medical devices, including endoluminal stents, distraction rods for scoliosis correction, mesh prostheses for laparoscopic hernioplasty, and bone staples.[39] Nitinol bone staples are generally prechilled, opened, and inserted into predrilled holes. The staple recovers either by application of an external energy source or by body temperature to pull the bone ends together. There

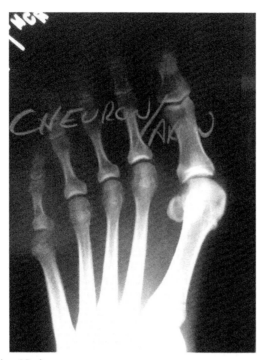

Fig. 12. Preoperative AP view.

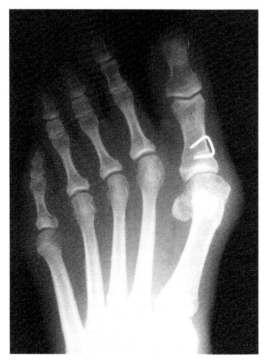

Fig. 13. AP view showing Akin osteotomy using bone staples.

are 3 types of commercially available staples: room-temperature superelastic, body-temperature activated, and heat activated.[43] Of the various commercially available types of shape memory staples, the different staple types have different procedural characteristics and inherent compressive forces. It has been shown that the heat-activated staples achieved the best balance of high fixation forces and procedural control. By contrast, the lowest compressive forces were consistently seen in the body-temperature activated staples.[43]

In a biochemical study by Farr and colleagues,[41] the investigators compared shape memory compression staples and mechanical compression staples. The effect of altering staple limb length was also assessed. It was found that the limbs of all mechanical compression staples diverged, causing inconsistent compression and distraction. The shape memory staples all achieved consistent compression across the fusion site and consistently greater compressive forces as compared with the mechanical compression staples. Also, staple limb length did not alter the compressive force generated.

Shibuya and colleagues[44] performed a biomechanical study of 3 different staples in calcaneal bone models. After comparing the ability of the OSStaple (BioMedical Enterprises Inc, San Antonio, TX, USA), UNI-CLIP (Newdeal Inc, USA, Plano, TX, USA) and Smith and Nephew Standard Large Staple (Smith & Nephew Inc, Memphis, TN, USA) to maintain compression, the investigators found that the OSStaple consistently generated the greatest and most uniform compression. In addition, the OSStaple sustained the compression the longest over the duration of the trials. In a similar study involving the Richards staple (Smith and Nephew Inc, Memphis, TN, USA), it was found to be 4 times stiffer in both bending and torsional forces than the memory staples, using bone models. However, the Richards staple was shown to have permanent deformation after the force was removed.[45]

Mereau and Ford[39] performed a retrospective study in patients who underwent an arthrodesis or an osteotomy fixated using the shape memory staples OSStaples and Memodyn staples (Telos Medical, Fallston, MD, USA). Fifteen Akin osteotomies were performed, 8 using OSStaple and 7 using the Memodyn staple, and were fixated using either one or two staples. In all cases, the lateral cortex of the osteotomy site was left intact. In 2 of the cases with the OSStaple, the lateral cortex fractured 6 and 10 weeks after surgery, the fixation appeared stable radiographically, and healed at 9 and 14 weeks. In both of those cases only a single staple was inserted from medial to lateral, engaging only the medial cortex. In 2 of the cases using the Memodyn staple, there was malposition of the osteotomy deemed unrelated to the fixation. The investigators concluded that compression staples provided an excellent source of internal fixation, and were technically easier to use and with fewer steps than AO applied screws. It was found that fixation effectiveness is increased by a greater number of staples, thus more than one staple was recommended. Regarding this point, a similar study showed 2 staples across an arthrodesis site yields the largest proportional increase in torsional stability when compared with single-screw or single-staple fixation.[46]

Malal and Kumar[47] used memory staples for fixation of 7 Akin osteotomies. In their study, staple back-out or displacement was not seen in any of the cases. These investigators suggested that the use of these staples may reduce the time to fusion and healing, reducing the recovery time following surgery.

Bioabsorbable devices are alternatives for internal fixation of fractures, osteotomies, and arthrodesis. Many compounds are bioabsorbable; however, only a few possess the required properties necessary for internal fixation. The most commonly used materials are PGA, PLA, PLLA, and PDS (polyglycolide, polylactide, polylevolactic acid, and polydioxanone, respectively).[48] Bioabsorbable fixation attempts to limit complications by allowing a gradual transfer of stress forces on the newly forming bone, prevents atrophy of the surrounding bone due to a lack of functional stimuli, and avoids further surgical procedures for removal of other forms of internal fixation.[49]

Barca and Busa[49] performed a total of 25 Akin osteotomies using either one or two PLLA BIO-R-SORB mini-staples with an average follow-up of 16 months. The average time of union of the osteotomies was approximately 4 weeks. No significant difference in healing times was observed in patients treated with one or two bioabsorbable staples. Neither pseudoarthrosis, malunion or nonunion, nor breakage of the staples were seen in any of the cases. The investigators concluded that considering the high rate of subjective and objective results, they encourage the use of the PLLA bioabsorbable staples, which can be used as an alternative to traditional nonabsorbable types for fixation of Akin osteotomies.

With the recent advances in metal alloy engineering and bioabsorbable materials, the fixation of Akin osteotomies with shape memory staples and bioabsorbable staples is a viable alternative to other forms of fixation. According to investigators, nitinol compression staples are technically easier, with fewer steps than AO applied screws, and provide comparable fixation for arthrodesis and osteotomies of the foot, including Akin osteotomies.[39]

SUMMARY

Implant technologies are allowing innovative bunion correction techniques. The OBW plate allows stable fixation of an inherently unstable osteotomy. The powerful corrective ability of the OBW osteotomy will see resurgence in the coming years. Similarly, the locked plating for the Lapidus allows for earlier weight bearing and will gain favor with patients and surgeons alike. TightRope use in bunion correction is not without its complications; however, as techniques and utilization advance, select patients may benefit from its use. The use of a staple for the Akin offers another viable option as fixation techniques are evaluated. Overall, more options are available to surgeons for bunion correction than ever before. Procedure-specific implants are allowing precise fixation to improve outcomes when performing bunion correction.

REFERENCES

1. Trethowan J. Hallux valgus. In: Choyce CC, editor. A system of surgery. New York: Hoeber, PG; 1923. p. 1046–9.
2. Hardy MA, Grove JR. Opening base wedge osteotomy of the first metatarsal using the Arthrex low profile plate and screw system. The Foot and Ankle Online Journal 2009;2(4).
3. Randhawa S, Pepper D. Radiographic evaluation of hallux valgus treated with opening wedge osteotomy. Foot Ankle Int 2009;30(5):427–31.
4. Wukich DK, Roussel AJ, Dial DM. Correction of metatarsus primus varus with an opening wedge plate: a review of 18 procedures. J Foot Ankle Surg 2009;48(4): 420–6.
5. Saragas NP. Proximal opening-wedge osteotomy of the first metatarsal for hallux valgus using a low profile plate. Foot Ankle Int 2009;30(10):976–80.
6. Shurnas PS, Watson TS, Crislip TW. Proximal first metatarsal opening wedge osteotomy with a low profile plate. Foot Ankle Int 2009;30(9):865–72.
7. Cooper MT, Berlet GC, Shurnas PS, et al. Proximal opening-wedge osteotomy of the first metatarsal for correction of hallux valgus. Surg Technol Int 2007;16: 215–9.

8. Wukich DK, Roussel AJ, Dial DM. Opening wedge osteotomy of the first metatarsal base: a technique for correction of metatarsal primus varus using a new titanium opening wedge plate. Oper Tech Orthop 2006;16(1):76–81.

9. Smith WB, Hyer CF, DeCarbo WT, et al. Opening wedge osteotomies for correction of hallux valgus: a review of wedge plate fixation. Foot Ankle Spec 2009;2(6): 277–82.

10. Lapidus PW. Operative correction of metatarsus varus primus in hallux valgus. Surg Gynecol Obstet 1934;58:183–91.

11. Cotzee JC, Resig SG, Kuskowski M. The Lapidus procedure as salvage after failed surgical treatment of hallux valgus: a prospective cohort study. J Bone Joint Surg Am 2003;85:60–5.

12. Fuhrmann RA. Arthrodesis of the first tarsometatarsal joint for correction of the advanced splayfoot accompanied by a hallux valgus. Oper Orthop Traumatol 2005;17:195–210.

13. Myerson M, Allon S, McGarvey W. Metatarsocuneiform arthrodesis for management of hallux valgus and metatarsus primus varus. Foot Ankle 1992;13:107–15.

14. Saffo G, Wooster MF, Stevens M, et al. First metatarsocuneiform joint arthrodesis: a five-year retrospective analysis. J Foot Surg 1989;28:459–65.

15. Sangeorzan BJ, Hansen ST Jr. Modified Lapidus procedure for hallux valgus. Foot Ankle 1989;9:262–6.

16. Cohen DA, Parks BG, Schon LC. Screw fixation compared to H-locking plate fixation for first metatarsocuneiform arthrodesis: a biomechanical study. Foot Ankle Int 2005;26:984–9.

17. Gruber F, Sinkov VS, Bae SY, et al. Crossed screws versus dorsomedial locking plate with compression screw for first metatarsocuneiform arthrodesis: a cadaver study. Foot Ankle Int 2008;29(9):927–30.

18. Marks RM, Parks BG, Schon LC. Midfoot fusion technique for neuropathic feet: biomechanical analysis and rationale. Foot Ankle Int 1998;12:507–10.

19. Scranton PE, Coetzee JC, Carreira D. Arthrodesis of the first metatarsocuneiform joint: a comparative study of fixation methods. Foot Ankle Int 2009;30(4): 341–5.

20. Saxena A, Nguyen A, Nelsen E. Lapidus bunionectomy: early evaluation of crossed lag screw versus locking plate with plantar lag screw. J Foot Ankle Surg 2009;48(2):170–9.

21. Sorensen MD, Hyer CF, Berlet GC. Results of Lapidus arthrodesis and locked plating with early weight bearing. Foot Ankle Spec 2009;2(5):227–33.

22. Walz L, Salzmann GM, Fabbro T, et al. The anatomic reconstruction of acromioclavicular joint dislocations using 2 TightRope devices: a biomechanical study. Am J Sports Med 2008;36(12):2398–406.

23. Cottom JM, Hyer CF, Philbin TM, et al. Treatment of syndesmotic disruptions with the Arthrex Tightrope: a report of 25 cases. Foot Ankle Int 2008;29(8):773–80.

24. Shrum DG. Ligamentation of the adductor hallucis tendon in bunionectomy. J Am Podiatr Med Assoc 2002;92(9):512–51.

25. Ponnapula P, Wittock R. Application of an interosseous suture and button device for hallux valgus correction: a review of outcomes in a small series. J Foot Ankle Surg 2010;49(2):159.e21–2.

26. Holmes GB Jr. Correction of hallux valgus deformity using the Mini TightRope device. Tech Foot Ankle Surg 2008;7(1):9–16.

27. Comprehensive solutions for forefoot and midfoot surgery using the Mini TightRope system. Five surgical techniques. Copyright. Naples (FL): Arthrex Inc; 2008. All rights reserved. LB0004A.

28. West BC. Mini TightRope system for hallux abducto valgus deformity: a discussion and case report. J Am Podiatr Med Assoc 2010;100(4):291–5.
29. Laughlin TJ. Complications of distal first metatarsal osteotomies. J Foot Ankle Surg 1995;34(6):524–31.
30. Kemp TJ, Hirose CB, Coughlin MJ. Fracture of the second metatarsal following suture button fixation device in the correction of hallux valgus. Foot Ankle Int 2010;31(8):712–6.
31. Mader DW, Han NM. Bilateral second metatarsal stress fractures after hallux valgus correction with the use of a tension wire and button fixation system. J Foot Ankle Surg 2010;49(5):488.e15–9.
32. Arthrex Research and Development. The effect of tunnel placement in the 2nd metatarsal on the ultimate strength of the 2nd metatarsal after hallux valgus correction using the TightRope system. Copyright. Arthrex Inc; 2008. All rights reserved. LA0439A.
33. Akin OF. The treatment of hallux valgus: a new operative procedure and its results. Med Sentinel 1925;33:678–9.
34. Mitchell LA, Baxter DE. A Chevron-Akin double osteotomy for correction of hallux valgus. Foot Ankle 1991;12(1):7–14.
35. Roukis TS. Hallux proximal phalanx Akin-Scarf osteotomy. J Am Podiatr Med Assoc 2004;94(1):70–2.
36. Sabo D. Correction osteotomy of the first phalanx of the great toe (Akin osteotomy). Int Surg 2007;2:66–9.
37. Langford JH. ASIF Akin osteotomy: a new method of fixation. J Am Podiatry Assoc 1981;71(7):390–6.
38. Murphy JS, Mozena JD, Walker RE. Kwire technique for fixation of the Akin osteotomy. J Am Podiatr Med Assoc 1989;79(6):291–3.
39. Mereau TM, Ford TC. Nitinol compression staples for bone fixation in foot surgery. J Am Podiatr Med Assoc 2006;96(2):102–6.
40. Ostgaard HC, Ebel P, Irstam L. Fixation of ankle fractures: power-driven staples compared with a routine method, a 3-year follow-up study. J Orthop Trauma 1990;4(4):415–9.
41. Farr D, Karim A, Lutz M. A biomechanical comparison of shape memory compression staples and mechanical compression staples: compression or distraction? Knee Surg Sports Traumatol Arthrosc 2010;18(2):212–7.
42. Buehler WJ. WOL oral history supplement. NITINOL Re-examination. WOLAA LEAF. 2006. vol. 8:1 [newsletter].
43. Russel SM. Design considerations for nitinol bone staples. J Mater Eng Perform 2009;18(5–6):831–5.
44. Shibuya N, Manning SN, Mezzaros A, et al. A compression force comparison study among three staple fixation systems. J Foot Ankle Surg 2007;46(1):7–15.
45. Rethnam U, Kuiper J, Makwana N. Mechanical characteristics of three staples commonly used in foot surgery. J Foot Ankle Res 2009;2(5) [online].
46. Bechtold JE, Meidt JD, Varecka TF, et al. The effect of staple size, orientation, and number on torsional fracture fixation stability. Clin Orthop 1993;297:210–7.
47. Malal JJG, Kumar CS. The use of memory(R) staples in foot and ankle surgery. J Bone Joint Surg Br 2008;90(Suppl II):231.
48. Rokkanen PU, Bostman O, Hirvensalo E, et al. Bioabsorbable fixation in orthopaedic surgery and traumatology. Biomaterials 2000;21(24):2607–13.
49. Barca F, Busa R. Resorbable poly-L-lactic acid mini-staples for the fixation of Akin osteotomies. J Foot Ankle Surg 1997;36(2):106–11.

The Cheilectomy and its Modifications

Molly Schnirring-Judge, DPM[a,b,c,d,*], Dave Hehemann, DPM[e]

KEYWORDS

- Hallux limitus • Hallux rigidus • Modified cheilectomy
- Dorsiflexory wedge osteotomy

Depending on the age group of assessed adults, middle-age women, or the elderly, hallux abducto valgus (HAV) deformity has been reported to represent as much as 33%, 38%, and 70% of the population, respectively.[1–3] Meanwhile hallux rigidus may represent only as much as 10% of persons aged 20 to 34 years but as much as 44% of people older than 80 years.[4,5] Despite the fact that hallux rigidus is less prevalent it does result in significant impairment and pain and so has a very important negative impact on function.[6] In considering the elderly this dysfunction and pain is suspected to increase the risk of falling. If not for this reason alone it is important to understand the nature of degenerative joint disease as it affects the 1st metatarsal phalangeal joint (MTPJ) and how it disrupts the normal ability to bear weight and propulse of the great toe joint. Due to the severity of the impairment that this condition can cause, surgical intervention has been suggested for cases that have failed conservative methods. The modified cheilectomy is considered by many the first-line treatment for this disease, given the procedure's inherent ability to eliminate degenerate bone and cartilage, decompressing the intra-articular space, while sparing cubic content of bone.[7–10] Once the cheilectomy has been performed, there remains a sufficient volume of bone to perform a more definitive reconstruction, such as an arthrodesis of the first metatarsophalangeal joint, should that ever be required.[11,12] The modified cheilectomy has proven to be an effective, efficient, inexpensive and conservative method that improves 1st MTPJ function with predictable outcomes in appropriate candidates.

[a] Publications and Research, Cleveland Clinic Foundation-Kaiser Permanente Foundation Podiatric Residency Program, Cleveland, OH, USA
[b] Colleges of Podiatric Medicine and Ohio University, Athens, OH, USA
[c] Graduate Medical Education, Mercy Health Partners, Toledo, OH, USA
[d] Private Practice, North West Ohio Foot and Ankle Institute LLC, Serving Ohio and Michigan, Lambertville, MI, USA
[e] Cleveland Clinic Foundation-Kaiser Permanente, Cleveland, OH, USA
* Corresponding author. Publications and Research, Cleveland Clinic Foundation-Kaiser Permanente Foundation Podiatric Residency Program, Cleveland, OH.
E-mail address: mjudgemolly@aim.com

Clin Podiatr Med Surg 28 (2011) 305–327
doi:10.1016/j.cpm.2011.03.004
0891-8422/11/$ – see front matter © 2011 Elsevier Inc. All rights reserved.

podiatric.theclinics.com

HISTORICAL REVIEW

In 1887 Davies-Colley coined the term *hallux flexus* in defining the degenerative condition of the great toe resulting in stiffness and swelling of the first MTPJ.[13] Cotterill would later lay claim to the term *hallux rigidus* for pain associated with attempted dorsiflexion of the phalanx on the first metatarsal.[14] It is presumed that these conditions actually represent 2 phases of the same process involving injury, chronic inflammation, and degenerative change of the chondral surface and underlying subchondral bone that yields progressive joint restriction and chronic pain. The condition likened to osteochondritis desiccans is a wearing process that results in cartilage degeneration and ultimately eburation of subchondral bone.

As the condition was reported more frequently, the mechanics of the condition became a source of discussion and debate. In 1895 the term *hallux dolorosus* was proposed by Walsham and Hughes, given the Latin adjective meaning intensely sad or painful.[15] In 1937 Hiss described this joint restriction as *hallux limitus* and that term is most commonly used today. In the following year Lambrinudi coined the term metatarsus primus elevatus, and described its ability to contribute to hallux rigidus. The mechanics of this structural deformity; an elevated position of the first metatarsal and hallux equinus, are commonly understood and are believed to incite this chronic degenerative joint disease. Lapidus introduced the term dorsal bunion in 1940. Despite the multitude of terms used to describe arthritis and decreased motion of the first MTPJ, *hallux limitus* and *hallux rigidus* remain the most commonly used in the current literature.

ETIOLOGY OF HALLUX LIMITUS/HALLUX RIGIDUS

Regarding the ultimate culprit for hallux limitus and hallux rigidus, the senior author (M.S.J.) subscribes to an early description of the disease provided by Goodfellow,[16] who relates the condition to osteochondritis desiccans. The precursor of this condition is not readily apparent on plain radiographs, and not until the condition undergoes repair is the evidence of prior damage and disease revealed. It can be extrapolated from this that the chronic inflammation associated with repair causes fibrosis of the soft tissue structures of the joint periphery and so capsular adhesion, sesamoid degenerative change, and fibrosis contribute to joint restriction as a consequence. Although there are multiple biomechanical factors thought to contribute to the development of hallux rigidus, the pathology that progresses subsequent to joint damage, whether it be acute injury or chronic wear from repetitive cyclic loading, most closely approximates the dysvascular and progressively degenerative change of osteochondritis desiccans. Nilsonne[17] defined primary and secondary hallux rigidus subtypes to annotate the epidemiology of the disease. The term *primary* hallux rigidus described the condition with adolescent onset, whereas *secondary* hallux rigidus was described as an adult variety that is chronic and long-standing. Further, the condition can be subdivided into *functional hallux limitus* (weight bearing) and *structural hallux limitus* (non–weight bearing). It is suggested that functional hallux limitus is associated with an uncompensated forefoot varus with or without hallux equinus. Often a contracture of the extensor hallucis longus is a concomitant finding. By contrast, structural hallux limitus is associated with an elevated first metatarsal. The nature of hallux equinus has been correlated with first MTPJ limitation, and consequently primary and secondary hallux equinus has been described. Primary hallux equinus is associated with flexible forefoot varus and muscular spasticity, whereas secondary hallux equinus is associated with metatarsal equinus and uncompensated forefoot varus.[18]

The following are some of the more common structural conditions suggested as a cause of hallux limitus/rigidus: short or long first metatarsal, elevated first metatarsal (iatrogenic or congenital), flat foot, osteoarthritis of the sesamoid apparatus, hypermobile first ray, metabolic conditions (eg, rheumatoid arthritis and gout), and acute and repetitive trauma.[15,17,19–27] The cause of this joint restriction is commonly multifactorial, and includes physical factors such as age, habitus, shoe gear, activities of daily living, trauma, and family history of osteoarthritis. In 2002 Grady and colleagues[28] retrospectively reviewed 772 patients treated for hallux rigidus. Of these patients, 43% had more than one contributing factor and 55% were associated with trauma.

CLASSIFICATION OF HALLUX LIMITUS/HALLUX RIGIDUS

Although the precise etiology of this condition remains obscure, the focus of practitioners remains in the diagnosis and treatment of the disease. Classification systems developed over time are numerous; however, the most useful of these provide a means to correlate clinical and radiographic findings with potential treatment options.

In 1986 Regnauld[29] developed and reported a classification system based on clinical findings and radiographic deformity of the first MTPJ, and this has remained popular for decades. In this system, first-degree through third-degree hallux rigidus defines the progression of pain and joint limitation along with the tell-tale radiographic changes that affect the joint and sesamoid apparatus. First-degree hallux rigidus includes the clinical findings of pain at end range of motion (ROM) with 40° of dorsiflexion and 20° of plantar flexion, while on plain radiographs there is slight narrowing of the joint space with loss of the normal convexity of the metatarsal head mirroring the loss of the phalangeal base concavity. Evidence of generalized forefoot osteopenia and slight sesamoid hypertrophy are also noted. Second-degree hallux rigidus reveals more important clinical changes, such as intermittent pain that may be noticed on and off weight bearing, with more significant limitation of joint motion and noticeable loss of suppleness in adjacent soft tissues. A dorsal exostosis is associated with this phase of the disease, and a noticeable hygroma or cystic-type swelling about the plantar joint soft tissues may become apparent. With derangement of the joint, lateral transfer of load, resulting in lesser metatarsalgia and discomfort from compensations affecting the Lis Franc joint complex, evolves. On radiography there is continued narrowing of joint space, flattening of the metatarsal head with osteophytic borders, and hypertrophy of the sesamoids. Eburnation of the metatarsal head is evidenced by loss of the metatarsal head contours, including flattening of the central aspect with an associated fine sclerotic rim as evidence of the bone impaction and hardening. Finally, in the third degree joint limitation becomes incapacitating, and extensive spurring and ankylosis of the parts are associated with bone bossing. Regnauld described a loss of joint pain in third-degree hallux rigidus, due to the immobility of the MTPJ; this could be associated with sesamoid hypertrophy, causing contracture and traction at the phalangeal base with distortion of its normal morphology. Contracture of the flexor hallucis longus results in plantar keratosis beneath the hallux interphalangeal joint, and the foot assumes a varus configuration. Pain in third-degree hallux rigidus was felt to be caused by neuritis within the first intermetatarsal space and dorsal exostosis, with bursal formations at risk for ulceration.[29] More recent updated classification schemes have been developed and discussed over time; however, none have successfully correlated clinical and radiographic findings with intraoperative findings.[30–34] Coughlin and Shurnas[30,31,33] developed a 5-stage classification after following patients for a 19-year period. Their classification consists of both radiographic and clinical findings for which grades 1 to 3 are very similar to Regnauld's classification, but include more detailed descriptions of dorsiflexory capacity of the joint. In this system grade 0 indicates dorsiflexion of 40° to 60° with stiffness and/or restriction of 10% to 20% (compared with the contralateral limb) and stage 4, which is equivalent to Regnaulds 3rd degree has the addition of pain at mid ROM. The importance of this classification system is that it correlates the dorsiflexion capacity of the joint with the severity of the condition.

Roukis and colleagues[34] further developed a 4-stage radiographic classification as an off-shoot of the Coughlin classification, whereby grade IV takes into consideration degenerative changes within the first and second metatarsal cuneiform joints.

CONSIDERATIONS IN CONSERVATIVE MANAGEMENT

Regardless of the classification system used or the grade assigned to patients, the condition should be treated conservatively to failure. Conservative measures often include oral or topical nonsteroidal anti-inflammatories, orthoses modified with Morton's extension, shoe gear modifications (rocker sole shoe, metatarsal roll bar, and so forth), and lifestyle and activity modifications. Whereas some contend that intra-articular steroid injections have a role in the conservative treatment of hallux limitus/rigidus, given its anti-inflammatory effect the senior author does not subscribe to this method as it can carry potential side effects that risk higher degrees of morbidity should the adjacent capsular and tendinous structures undergo attenuation or rupture subsequent to steroid exposure. In the category of supplemental therapy more recent consideration includes the use of injected hyaluronate sodium, a viscous solution touted to slow down, if not halt, the progression of the degenerative disease and to encourage healing. The viscoelastic properties of this solution provide mechanical protection for tissues by providing a shock-absorbing buffer, and facilitate wound healing. Hyaluronate sodium is believed to facilitate transport of peptide growth factors to a site of action. Once at the site the hyaluronan is degraded and active proteins are released, promoting tissue repair. To date this therapy is considered as a last stage in conservative therapy, and has been used for conditions including hallux rigidus, stenosing tenosynovitis, and osteoarthritis of the knee and ankle joints among others. Of note, there are published reactions associated with this sodium salt of hyaluronan, and these reactions for the most part seem to be well localized and include injection site pain or rash, pruritus, headache, joint swelling, and joint effusion. This agent, however, does not carry the potential ill effects that long-acting steroids impose. For example, the published potential side effects of triamcinolone acetanide are numerous and include musculoskeletal reactions such as aseptic necrosis, Charcot-like arthropathy, calcinosis, muscle weakness, steroid-induced myopathy, tendon rupture, osteoporosis, and pathologic fracture, to mention but a few. Other adverse reactions are possible and may be even more severe depending on the location, dosage applied, and frequency of injections. Perhaps the most commonly discussed ill effects of steroid compounds are their potential to blunt the natural immune response, dermal and soft tissue atrophy, and increased risk of infection.

Another method that would seem to be a more physiologic approach to joint supplementation is the use of autologous platelet-derived growth factor (PDGF) application; however, such has not been borne out of the current literature. Given the notion that PDGF has the potential to stimulate if not enhance the healing process, it seems intuitive that this would promote a healthier environment for bone and cartilage as opposed to intra-articular steroid application, which is considered the more traditional approach. Although the use of PDGF would not be considered curative, it does carry the potential to stimulate a cellular response that is believed to be beneficial to both bone and joint health.

SURGICAL PROCEDURES FOR HALLUX LIMITUS/RIGIDUS

When conservative measures fail then surgery can be entertained, beginning with detailed patient education and informed consent. The corrective procedures designed for hallux limitus are as numerous as the terms used to describe the condition. Beginning in 1887, Davies and Colley proposed resection of the proximal half of the proximal phalanx. Collier[35] performed a first metatarsal head resection to decompress the joint. In 1927 Watermann described a resection of the dorsal spur combined with a dorsal wedge osteotomy to rotate the plantar cartilage dorsally. Multiple investigators beginning in the 1950s proposed fusion of the first MTPJ.[22,36,37] In 1958 Kessel and Bonney[38] performed a dorsal wedge resection on the base of the proximal phalanx. Throughout the years various investigators have promoted the use of the cheilectomy, a procedure that resects exostoses and recontours the joint to restore a ball and socket morphology to the joint, and several modifications have been advocated in the literature. Beginning in 1927, Cochrane[39] recommended an exostectomy, but was of the opinion that a plantar capsulotomy and incision to release the plantar intrinsic musculature at the base of the proximal phalanx was required. Later, Nilsonne[17] reported performing an exostectomy on 2 patients. He discontinued the surgical technique because of concern that the procedure did not provide a definitive result. Almost 30 years later, in 1959, DuVries[12] described in detail the surgical technique of the cheilectomy. He advocated that the cheilectomy should be the initial surgical treatment of choice for hallux rigidus. Since that time many investigators have advocated the use of cheilectomy for stage I and II hallux rigidus.[8,9,31–34,40–46]

In 1987 at a surgical seminar in Hershey, Pennsylvania, Valenti described a resection of bone from both the first metatarsal and the proximal phalanx. Within the last 20 years investigators have reported on modifications of the cheilectomy, but as yet few have attempted to document a direct correlation of these methods with functional outcome. Modifications include alteration to the incisional approach, subchondral drilling of cartilage defects, plantar capsule release, and dorsiflexory wedge osteotomy combined with a cheilectomy.[9,46–49] There has been widespread use of the cheilectomy despite one article's description of the ill effect of this technique on the biomechanics of the joint revealed in a cadaveric study. This study looked at 5 cadaveric specimens (10 feet) and evaluated the effects of the first MTPJ cheilectomy, and described abnormal compression created across the residual metatarsal head cartilage due to the altered morphology and function of the first MTPJ.[50] It is interesting to note that some of the best articles written on the use of the modified cheilectomy appeared after this experiment was published.[11,30,31,33,41,43,51–53]

FUNDAMENTALS OF THE CHEILECTOMY

In 1979 Mann and colleagues[9] reviewed the cheilectomy as originally reported by DuVries. Aside from detailing DuVries' surgical technique, they reviewed the outcome for 20 patients who underwent cheilectomy. At an average of 67.6 months' follow-up, patients were capable of 30° of first MTPJ dorsiflexion on average. The investigators reported little or no progression of the degenerative process at the time of long-term follow-up. Subjectively there was "uniform" satisfaction among patients, ranging from 7 months to 156 months post procedure. This result suggests that early patient satisfaction after the cheilectomy does not seem to reduce over time, which is a powerful implication of this research. In 1988 Mann and Clanton[54] performed cheilectomies on

25 patients, with an average follow-up of 56 months. In this study a total of 31 procedures were reviewed. Twenty-two joints had complete relief. Six of the remaining joints had relief most of the time with an occasional episode of pain. Despite relatively small patient populations, these articles provide positive functional results in support of using the modified cheilectomy for joint salvage. These findings are consistent with a meta-analysis performed by Roukis[11] suggesting that the cheilectomy is a useful procedure appropriate as first-line surgical treatment for hallux rigidus, and has a low overall incidence of the need for revisional surgery.

Coughlin and Shurnas[31] further examined 110 patients with long-term follow-up of hallux rigidus treatment. Of these 110, 80 patients underwent cheilectomy. The mean follow-up for this group was 9.6 years. Patients treated by cheilectomy demonstrated significant improvement in ROM, pain, and American Orthopaedic Foot and Ankle Society (AOFAS) scores. Of note, the scoring and results did not correlate with radiographic appearance of the joint at time of follow-up. Of the 80 patients who underwent cheilectomies, 92% were considered successes. Most of the cheilectomies were performed on hallux rigidus grades I and II. In 9 patients with grade IV disease cheilectomy was performed and later, at an average of 6.9 years status post cheilectomy, underwent a first MTPJ arthrodesis.[31] It is important that the investigators did not recommend cheilectomy for patients with grade IV disease, so the failure of treatment in these 5 patients who ultimately required arthrodesis was not surprising.

Multiple other investigators have advocated that cheilectomy be reserved for hallux rigidus grades I and II. In 1986 Hattrup and Johnson[44] reported on 58 patients with hallux rigidus. Overall satisfaction was 53.4% of patients completely satisfied, 19% mostly satisfied, and 27.6% unsatisfied. Average follow-up for this study was 37 months. It was noted that with grade I hallux rigidus (Regnauld classification) there was 15% failure rate of the cheilectomy. With grades II and III a 31.8% and 37.5% failure rate, respectively, was noted. Similar to Hattrup and Johnson, in 1997 Mackay and colleagues[55] evaluated 34 patients with hallux rigidus and reported outcomes based on grade. Patients were evaluated on postoperative pain, activity levels, shoe gear, ability to walk on tiptoe, and ROM. Consistent with studies previously mentioned, patients with lower grades of hallux rigidus demonstrated the most improvement. Overall satisfactory outcome achieved for grades I, II, and III was 94%, 100%, and 66%, respectively. The investigators concluded that for grades I and II hallux limitus, cheilectomy should be the treatment of choice. This study had a small population for grade III; subsequently, the investigators could not make a definitive statement regarding that degree of disease and outcome following the cheilectomy procedure.

In considering the studies reviewed in the current literature it becomes apparent that surgical selection hinges on more than clinical and radiographic grade, and that other factors can affect decision making. Two factors affecting surgical selection are activity level and the age of the patient. In 1999 Mulier and colleagues[43] chose to evaluate the effects of cheilectomy on athletes with either Regnauld grade I or II hallux limitus. Cheilectomies were performed on 22 feet and evaluated at a mean 5-year follow-up. Patients were functionally graded postoperatively as 14 excellent, 7 good, and 1 fair. Thirteen patients were evaluated for longer than 4 years. Of these 13 patients, 7 had increasing radiographic changes despite good functional outcomes. Of the 22 patients, 75% returned to athletic activity at previous level or higher. Of note, the functional outcomes in 5 of the 7 remaining patients who did not return to previous athletic activity were not related to the surgery. The investigators concluded that cheilectomy is a viable option for an elite-level athlete.

Feltham and colleagues[8] reported on 67 patients receiving cheilectomies for hallux rigidus. Patients were evaluated using the Regnauld classification. The patients were then further subdivided by age. Overall 78% of the patients were satisfied with the cheilectomy at an average follow-up of 65-months. The investigators found no statistical correlation between the Regnauld classification and satisfaction rate. However, in patients older than 60 years there was a significantly higher satisfaction rate of 91%. Regardless of age and athletic ability, there was approximately an 80% to 90% success rate with the cheilectomy procedure. While outcomes may vary when considering age groups, athletic activity, and radiographic and clinical grade, there remains an advantage to using the cheilectomy, as it remains a joint salvage procedure that does not "burn any bridges" with regard to cubic content of bone available once the procedure has been performed.

Surgical approaches have varied since DuVries first described it. He described a dorsal incision. Two groups have attempted different incisional approaches and have examined whether they provide any benefits.

Lin and Murphy[45] examined 20 cheilectomies performed with a dorsal lateral approach versus the standard dorsal approach. The investigators' modification of the procedure employed an incision over the lateral edge of the first MTPJ. Cheilectomy was performed by removing the dorsal bump as well as osteophytes from the proximal phalanx. The most common complication was numbness in the first web space, which occurred in 40% of the patients. The average age of the patients was 53.8 years and the average follow-up was 2.8 years. At long-term follow-up there was a significant improvement in the clinical-radiographic staging. The patients' average AOFAS Score improved from 53.5 to 84. Age, increase in staging, and AOFAS score results were similar to other reports, and the investigators concluded that there was no advantage to the use of a lateral incision. By contrast, Easely and colleagues[41] explored using a medial approach to the cheilectomy in 68 feet with an average follow-up of 3 years. In addition to the dorsal cheilectomy, a plantar release was performed. The plantar release has been mentioned in passing in only few articles, and has never been directly compared with cheilectomies performed without a plantar release. Using the AOFAS scoring system the average improvement was from 45 to 85 points, with an increase in dorsiflexion and total ROM. The feet that were examined and treated were subdivided by grade. There were 17 grade I, 39 grade II, and 12 grade III feet. Of the 68 feet examined, 38 had worsened by at least one grade at follow-up. Of the 68 patients, 9 were symptomatic. Eight of the 9 symptomatic feet were grade III. The medial approach with a plantar release for a cheilectomy provides reliable results for hallux rigidus grades I and II, with less reliable results noted for grade III. The investigators noted that only 2 of the 12 grade III cheilectomies required fusion, in contrast to the Coughlin study. However, this may be due to the fact that the average follow-up was less than half that presented in the Coughlin report.[31] Alternately the fact that some cheilectomies seem to withstand the test of time while others do not may have to do with the ability of the surgeon to successfully eliminate degenerate bone. It stands to reason that degenerate bone will eventually succumb to the wear and tear process. This is especially true if abnormal biomechanics have been left unchecked post operatively.

Several investigators have studied the effects of cheilectomy on plantar pressures. Despite the fact that the cheilectomy does not surgically address deforming forces that may have caused the disease, it is hypothesized that plantar pressures would be restored with successful joint decompression. In 2008 Nawoczenski and colleagues[52] undertook an in vivo evaluation of the biomechanical affects of a cheilectomy. Twenty patients in the study were evaluated preoperatively, at 1.7 years and 6 years after the index procedure. At final evaluation only 15 patients were available, and it was found that the cheilectomy increased abduction and dorsiflexion at the first

MTPJ in all while reestablishing functional plantar pressures. Despite these improvements, the average increase in ROM and abduction was less than the required 45° necessary for daily activities. Further, it was noted that the hallux equinus remained essentially unchanged after the cheilectomy procedure, suggesting that the abnormal mechanics also remained unchanged.

CHEILECTOMY AND DORSIFLEXORY WEDGE OSTEOTOMY

A modification of the cheilectomy with the addition of a dorsiflexory wedge osteotomy was first reported by Desai and colleagues[47] as an alternative to joint-destructive procedures. An advantage to this modification is that it does not limit alternative surgical options if a revision becomes necessary. Recently, Roukis undertook a systematic review of the cheilectomy with dorsiflexory osteotomy of the proximal phalanx.[11] His search results and inclusion criteria took into consideration 11 studies. In this meta-analysis there was a total of 167 procedures performed with follow-up. Forty-one experienced complete relief, 108 had improvement in symptoms, and 18 were either unchanged or worse. Eighteen patients required revisional surgeries. Six of the 11 studies included in the review listed the number of procedures performed and at what grade. For grades I, II, and III there were 18, 128, and 31 procedures performed, respectively. Unfortunately, there were multiple variables addressed within the 11 studies reviewed. Because of the multiple variables, Roukis concluded that it was difficult to ascertain the corrections that provided relief. Some of the variables included biplanar osteotomy to correct hallux interphalangeous, difference between grading scales used, omission of dorsiflexory osteotomy unless 70° dorsiflexion or less was gained from cheilectomy, and differences in the adjunctive procedures performed. Despite the multiple variables identified, there was only a 4.8% surgical revision rate. By comparison, systematic reviews for the traditional cheilectomy/dorsiflexory osteotomy and the Valenti procedure had an 8.8% and 4.6% surgical revisional rate, respectively.

CHEILECTOMY AND MICROFRACTURE

Further modifications include the addition of subchondral drilling of the first metatarsal head, and this procedure and its outcomes were discussed in two articles.[46,48] The first article, published in 2004, focused on the technique of cheilectomy with the addition of a plantar release and microfracture of the metatarsal head using a dorsal medial approach to gain access to the joint. Approximately 25% of the head was resected using an oscillating saw in this technique. Next the plantar structures were freed with a McGlamry elevator; attention was paid to release the plantar capsule and insertion of the short flexor muscles on the proximal phalanx. Any cartilage lesions were then microfractured with an awl regardless of whether they were on the metatarsal head or the proximal phalanx. Thirty-seven cases of hallux limitus receiving treatment with this technique were reported.[46] The subsequent article, a prospective case series wherein 28 patients and 32 feet underwent the procedure of the combination of cheilectomy, plantar release, and the microfracture technique for the treatment of hallux rigidus, was published in 2005.[48] It is unclear whether there was an overlap between the clinical groups reported in these two articles. There was no comparison provided between their described technique and cheilectomy alone or cheilectomy combined with release of plantar structures. Using evaluation of radiographs and magnetic resonance imaging, 18 patients were classified as stage II and 14 as stage III according to Hattrup and Johnson.[44] Postoperatively the investigators noted a significant improvement in pain, function (an average increase of 19° of motion), and patient satisfaction at an average of 23 months' follow-up. Like most previous studies involving cheilec-tomy alone, poorer results were noted within patients classified as grade III hallux rigidus.

PEARLS IN PRACTICE USING THE MODIFIED CHEILECTOMY FOR HALLUX RIGIDUS

The senior author uses the modified cheilectomy as a primary tool for intervention in the case of hallux limitus or hallux rigidus that proves recalcitrant to conservative methods and interferes with a patient's quality of life (**Fig. 1**). The technique used was described by DuVries, and rarely includes adjunctive procedures. Over time this procedure has brought significant relief to patients suffering from joint restriction, pain and impairment imposed by either functional or structural hallux limitus.

The preoperative radiographic assessment includes standard dorsal plantar and lateral foot views in addition to special views; a stress lateral foot view to demonstrate the patient's functional capacity in weight bearing, and in some patients the forefoot axial view, obtained to best evaluate the condition of the cristae and the sesamoid apparatus (**Fig. 2**). Despite the preoperative effort made in classifying the stage of hallux rigidus, it is the contention of the senior author that the intraoperative findings continually prove to be more significant than anticipated from the clinical and radio-graphic classifications (**Figs. 3 and 4**).

Throughout the prospective series of surgeries detailed in the next section, the procedure of cheilectomy was performed essentially as described by DuVries.[12] The procedure is referred to as a modified cheilectomy, as the senior author per-formed this technique in a manner that excised diseased bone completely and did not simply restore the normal contours of the ball and socket of the first MTPJ. The bone resection consisted of removing the dorsal 1/4 to 1/3 of the 1st metatarsal head as dictated by the extent of the bone disease. A similar amount of bone was removed in some but not all cases. This procedure begins with an incision made dorsally at the mid shaft of the first metatarsal and extends distally beyond the mid shaft of the proximal phalanx. After dissecting down to the capsule, the extensor hallucis is identified, evaluated and then retracted and an incision is made through

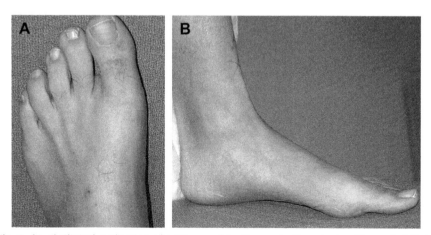

Fig. 1. (*A, B*) Clinical evaluation of a 42 year old active and otherwise healthy male fails to reveal outward signs of joint derangement. Specifically no hypertrophic bone formation, dorsal exostosis, bursal projections or evidence of dermal atrophy are seen in either the dorsal (*A*) or lateral (*B*) projections as seen here.

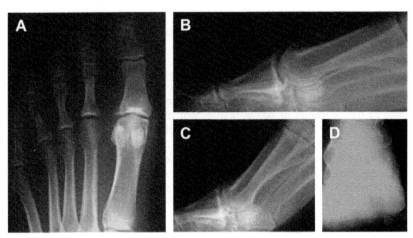

Fig. 2. (*A*) At first blush this dorsal plantar view is not very impressive although it demonstrates joint space narrowing with lateral joint lipping and subchondral cyst degeneration most impressive laterally. The sesamoids are squaring off however the joint and the position of the sesamoid apparatus remains congruous. (*B*) The lateral radiograph reveals the dorsal osteophytes and plantar joint narrowing. Overall this radiograph is not that impressive and in fact is out of proportion with the clinical complaint and the functional restriction in this patient. (*C*) Pre operative stress lateral view reveals the joint impingement and accentuates the morphologic changes that have affected the intra articular components of the joint. Notice the irregularity of the distal margin of the metatarsal head and the sclerotic margin at the base of the phalanx. The dorsal osteophytic lipping of both joint interfaces is commensurate with the subtle clinical fullness noted in the clinical evaluation. (*D*) The fore foot axial view reveals the position of the sesamoids, the condition of the cristae and the joint space between them. Notice that the sesamoids are not degenerative in this case and in fact are in a congruous position beneath the metatarsal head. Any virtual deviation of the sesamoids is the result of metatarsus primus varus and overall fore foot varus present in this patient.

the capsule in the same manner and length as the skin incision (see **Fig. 3**A). Plantarflexion with traction on the proximal phalanx is performed to best visualize the first metatarsal head (see **Fig. 3**B). Excision of the exostosis is performed dorsal, medial, and lateral about the joint (see **Fig. 3**C); a traditional cheilectomy restoring the normal rounded contour to the first MTPJ. The traditional procedure is modified to resect enough bone to double the range of dorsiflexion that was evident in the preoperative clinical assessment (and typically more). Care is taken as the dorsal metatarsal head is resected ensuring that the central and plantar cartilage is spared and that the sesamoid apparatus is not violated. Once the modified cheilectomy is complete the texture of the medial metatarsal head can be appreciated and appears much less porous as it is comprised of more densely compact bone after debridement. A deliberate effort is made to avoid excessive debridement about the interface of the metaphaseal-diaphyseal regions as aggressive resection here will increase the risk of post operative capsular adhesions. The base of the proximal phalanx is debrided to match the contour of the metatarsal head to create a congruous unit. Once adequate bone is resected (typically one-fourth to one-third of the metatarsal head), both joint surfaces are recontoured with a rasp (see **Fig. 3**D and E). Postoperatively the patient is allowed passive ROM when it becomes tolerable, usually within the first week after surgery.

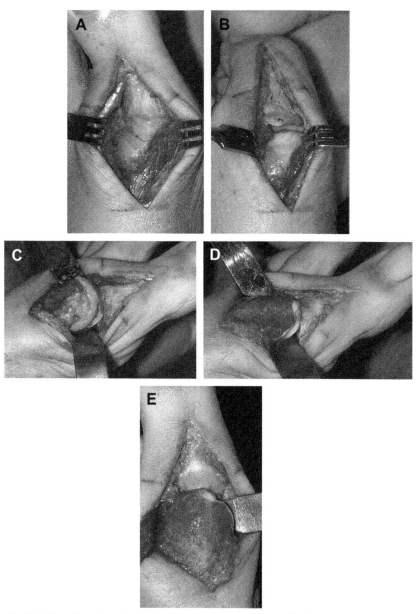

Fig. 3. (*A*) After dissecting down to the capsule, the extensor hallucis is retracted laterally and an incision made through the capsule of the same length as the skin incision. (*B*) Distraction and plantar flexion of the proximal phalanx is performed to aid in visualization of the first metatarsal head. Notice the bizarre morphology of the hypertrophic dorsal osteophyte extending laterally from the centroid of the 1st metatarsal head. (*C*) Excision of the exostosis is performed dorsal, medial, and lateral about the joint; a traditional cheilectomy restoring the normal rounded contour to the first MTPJ. (*D*) The traditional cheilectomy procedure is modified to resect enough bone to double the range of dorsiflexion that was evident in the preoperative clinical assessment (and typically more). Once adequate bone is resected (typically one-fourth to one-third of the metatarsal head), both joint surfaces are recontoured with a rasp. (*E*) The dorsal view, with the hallux superiorly in the field of view, reveals that all of the diseases bone has been resected and the underlying bone is of normal quality with porous bleeding smoothed surfaces.

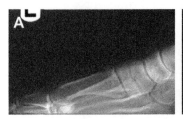
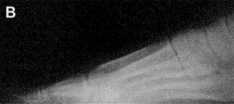

Fig. 4. Notice in these serial radiographs, (*A*) 4-weeks compared to (*B*) 6-months, that the 1st ray alignment is significantly different. In this earlier view (*A*) the 1st metatarsal is slightly elevated as evidenced by the divergence of the cortical margins of the 1st and 2nd metatarsal shafts. This is a reflection of a protected weight bearing posture as this patient progressed through a transient sesamoiditis. In the 6-month view (*B*) the sesamoiditis has been resolved and the dorsal cortex of the 1st metatarsal appears parallel to the 2nd as the 1st MTPJ is fully weight bearing without lateral load transfer.

POST OPERATIVE COURSE

Preoperative training for the use of an ortho wedge (heel weight-bearing) shoe is provided, and limited ambulation is allowed on the first postoperative day. After 2 weeks sutures are removed, and the patient is typically placed into a short leg-compression stocking once the incision is completely dry and well coapted. Serial radiographs are taken most typically at 2-weeks, 6-weeks, 10-weeks, 16-weeks and 24-weeks ensuring that the condition of the metatarsals remains unchanged over time (**Fig. 4**A, B). Given the fact that in many of these cases the 1st MTPJ has not been fully weight bearing in years it is prudent to monitor closely for early evidence of cortical hypertrophy, periostitis or resorptive changes as any of these may be harbingers of stress fracture or infection (see **Fig. 4**). Passive ROM exercises are performed throughout the early postoperative period, usually the first 10 days to 2 weeks, and active ROM exercises are performed thereafter as tolerated. The patient is instructed on in-home exercise; by simply sitting in a chair with the foot flat on the floor and then raising the heel, the foot is forced through a roll-off maneuver dorsiflexing the first MTPJ with the weight of the leg on the foot. This action is performed while wearing a short leg-compression stocking on the affected limb. The stocking provides a mild degree of compression and support for the joint while allowing active stretching maneuvers about the joint. Using an exercise that allows the patient to sit improves the patient's ability to control the degree of stress placed through the joint and titrate the motion to tolerance without eliciting unusual discomfort or anxiety. The first MTPJ is dorsiflexed to a maximum as tolerated, and this position is sustained for 10 seconds (**Fig. 5**B). Once the sustained stretch is performed on the affected foot, the patient performs the same maneuver for the contralateral foot. This action demonstrates to the patient the full motion of the normal (baseline) first MTPJ and serves as an example of the functional goal. Once the patient understands and is competent to perform the active ROM exercise, he or she can advance to the more aggressive daily activities that are important to their quality of life. This titration of activities is advanced quickly in most patients, who are typically able to return to their usual firm-soled athletic shoe gear within the first 3 to 6 weeks. It is not uncommon for the more physically active patients to return to the majority of their usual daily activities within the first month after surgery (**Fig. 5**).

If there are social issues such as accrued personal time off work (often more time than the recovery period requires) or employee's compensation claims, then the

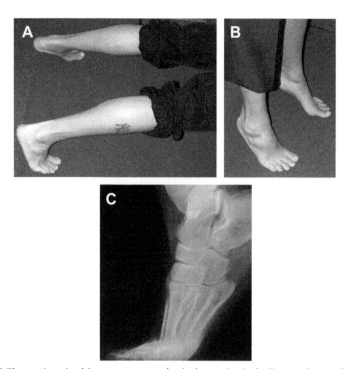

Fig. 5. (*A*) The patient is able to return to physical exercise including push ups that require end range dorsiflexion of the 1st MTPJ. The ability to perform this maneuver was in fact a key physical goal for this patient. (*B*) Bilateral toe rise ability depicted here has been restored to what the patient considers his "pre injury" condition. (*C*) The stress lateral view seen here is a long term follow up (6-year post op) evaluation demonstrating the ability to sustain a full weight bearing toe rise position. This far exceeds the pre operative joint restriction that was noted in (*C*).

time to full recovery is predictably longer. For this reason it is important to have a means of benchmarking the patient's function and subjective impression of his or her progress. **Fig. 6**A reveals the pre operative bench mark in full weight bearing dorsiflexion of the 1st MTPJ while (see **Fig. 6**B, C) depicts the pre operative radiographs demonstrating the stress lateral (see **Fig. 6**B) and position & alignment of the 1st MTPJ in the dorsal - plantar projection. Consequently, it is important to obtain the stress lateral radiograph in addition to standard radiograph views to demonstrate the radiographic and functional changes that have occurred since the time of surgery (see **Fig. 6**). Further, clinical survey forms are provided before surgery, within the first 8 weeks and periodically until final follow-up, to document the patient's own impression of the post operative progress. This process facilitates dialog between the patient and the surgeon and keeps the lines of communication open, allowing for continual discussion and question-and-answer sessions that are integral to the patient's overall satisfaction.

PROSPECTIVE CLINICAL DATA IN HALLUX LIMITUS AND HALLUX RIGIDUS

The following is a summary of a prospective study of 19 consecutive hallux limitus/hallux rigidus patients (21 feet) treated with the modified cheilectomy technique by

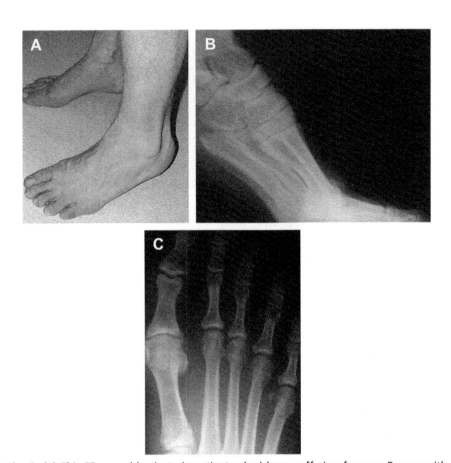

Fig. 6. (A) This 55-year old private investigator had been suffering for over 5-years with chronic pain and progressive loss of motion within the right great toe joint. He finally presented for treatment when he realized he couldn't tolerate running activities. (B) This pre operative stress lateral view reveals the end stage joint space narrowing and enlarged dorsal ostephytes with overlying bursal projection as evidenced by the focal soft tissue density. With close inspection the sesamoid joint can be identified and is narrowed. While a portion of the sesamoid apparatus is visible here this is not the optimal projection to assess the sesamoid apparatus. (C) This dorsal plantar view of the fore foot revelas the joint space narrowing and lateral osteophytes about the 1st MTPJ. Notice the joint remain congruous and that any abductus evident here is manifested distal to the MTPJ. The hypertrophic sesamoids are squared off and are only trace deviated on the midline of the metatarsal head.

the senior author. Exclusion criteria consisted of patients with diabetes, peripheral neuropathy, ulceration and infection of the foot or ankle. Ultimately no patients had to be excluded from the study. There were 10 females and 9 males, with 2 bilateral cases, both in females. Using the Regnauld classification system for hallux limitus there were 3 feet graded as Regnauld 1st degree, 15 2nd degree, and 3 3rd degree. For the 21 feet examined, the length pattern of the first metatarsal was evaluated on dorsal plantar radiographs. The first metatarsal length was assessed by measuring the length differential (in millimeters) by comparison of the centroid of the distal aspect of the first and second metatarsal heads. The first metatarsal was found to be shorter than the second metatarsal in 17 feet, longer than the second in 2, and equal to the second metatarsal in 2. There was no evidence of metatarsus primus elevatus in any patient entered into this study. Despite the majority of patient radiographs being assessed as a 2nd degree hallux limitus, the surgical inspection in each of the 21 feet revealed articular cartilage damage affecting 50% or more of the metatarsal head in addition to the peripheral hypertrophic bone and osteophytes about the medial, lateral, or both borders of the joint. In 13 of 21 feet there was subtle evidence of medial subluxation at the second MTPJ whereas only 5 of 21 of the second MTPJs were rectus. The chart of vital statistics from this patient series is shown in **Table 1**.

DISCUSSION ON THE UTILITY OF THE MODIFIED CHEILECTOMY

Although a specific etiology cannot be applied to every case of hallux limitus/rigidus, it is conceivable that this is a matter of an isolated osteochondritis identical to that seen elsewhere in the skeleton. The literature reveals numerous investigators discussing specific mechanics as the culprit for this condition; long or short first metatarsal, medial arch insufficiency, hypermobility of the first ray, and metatarsus primus elevatus, among others. If this disease is truly comprised of the spectrum of osteochondritis then early identification of this disease is the key to preventing it's progression and intervening as early as possible with joint-sparing orthotic devices should be the mainstay of therapy. This leaves the intense debate about the mechanics of the syndrome by the wayside. The mainstay then should be focused upon the orthotic prescription and addressing any structural or functional imbalances through that device. Should the orthotic plan fail then consideration for the modified cheilectomy is prudent. Further, in discussing the staging of this condition there has been an extensive amount

Table 1	
Prospective series of 21 cases of hallux limitus/hallux rigidus treated with the modified cheilectomy	
Number of patients: 19	Number of feet: 21
Gender: 10 females, 9 males	Two bilateral cases in female patients
Regnauld classification: Grade I: 3; Grade II: 15; Grade III: 3	
Second MTPJ position: 5 rectus, 13 medial subluxation, 3 lateral subluxation	
First metatarsal length: 17 shorter, 2 longer, 2 equal in length[a]	
Average age: 57.38 y	range: 41–70 y
Average follow-up reported: 85.9 wk	range: 4–270 wk
Preoperative American College of Foot and Ankle Surgeons (ACFAS) scoring system average: 45.08	range: 32–71
Postoperative ACFAS scoring system average: 76.57	range: 62–91
Preoperative VAS: 8.60	range: 5.00–10.00
Postoperative VAS: 1.38	post range: 0.00–7.00
Average percentage change in VAS score: 89.20	range: 30.00–100
Limp preoperatively: 17 patients	Limp postoperatively: 2 patients

Abbreviation: VAS, visual analog scale.
[a] First metatarsal length as compared with the second metatarsal length.

of literature supporting the belief that the stage of the disease is correlated with the development of an appropriate treatment plan. Current literature has delivered information on various groups of hallux limitus/rigidus patients that calls some of this dogma into question, specifically the difference between the clinical and radiographic grades of hallux rigidus as compared with the surgical grades of the disease. Although it may seem intuitive that the highest degrees of the condition would be associated with the worst outcomes, this correlation has not been borne out from the literature, nor has it been seen from the personal experience of the senior author in using the modified cheilectomy technique. In fact, the 4 patients who scored the lowest overall satisfaction in this study were associated with the development of sesamoiditis subsequent to noncompliance in orthotic therapy. Of these 4 patients, 2 were first-degree, 1 was second-degree, and one was third-degree hallux rigidus using the Regnauld classification scheme. This contradicts the typical notion correlating the classification and the outcome as 50% of these patients had the least significant form of the bone disease. In fact 75% of these patient's were considered of mild or moderate severity yet they were the least satisfied of the group.

Beyond this fact is that the utility of the modified cheilectomy has been supported by the medical literature since the 1920s when Cochrane described his approach that included release of plantar contractures of the long flexor and extrinsic musculature about the base of the phalanx. The technique of the cheilectomy, regardless of its modifications, was not truly embraced as a first-line therapy in the treatment of hallux rigidus until the 1950s. Since that time its utility for decompressing the joint and providing an improved ROM has been wholeheartedly supported by many.[7–9,40–45,51–62]

The senior author is among those who believe the modified cheilectomy, performed to eliminate degenerate bone and cartilage from the superior one-third of the joint, plays an important role in cases of severe and recalcitrant functional hallux limitus. In light of the joint decompression achieved by removal of this cubic content of bone, there is a virtual or functional lengthening of the dorsal soft tissue structures, which provides additional liberty to the joint. A cadaveric study of the change in motion vectors was undertaken comparing motion before and after cheilectomy of 30% and 50% of the metatarsal head diameter, which was found to improve the ROM in hallux rigidus specimens by 33%. Further, this study revealed that after cheilectomy, the proximal phalanx pivots rather than glides on the metatarsal head, yielding increased peak pressures at the end range of dorsiflexion and resulting in joint compression.[50] It is the senior author's contention that resection of the dorsal surfaces (modified cheilectomy) cannot be expected to restore normal gliding motion, as it merely decompresses the joint and leaves the the morphology of the metatarsal head grossly modified. In fact, hallux limitus and hallux rigidus conditions often equate to an irreversible change in the axis of motion about the first MTPJ. (Cases of metatarsus primus elevatus with first MTPJ dysfunction are an obvious exception, as this structural abnormality is able to be reversed in most circumstances.) For this reason the patient should be educated preoperatively that the modified cheilectomy does not change the abnormal mechanics that exist, but rather decompresses and relaxes dorsal joint structures, reducing intra-articular pressure and subsequently reduces pain with joint motion. Cochrane[39] originally described release of plantar contractures to improve function of the first MTPJ, and intuitively this is a reasonable consideration should the need for a plantar release become apparent intraoperatively. Hallux limitus is considered by some to be a condition limiting joint dorsiflexion to less than 65° (but more than 20°) and hallux rigidus as joint limitation less than 20° in total ROM at the first MTPJ.[63] In the prospective study reported herein, a majority of cases fell into the realm of hallux limitus from a clinical standpoint. It is interesting that despite the fact that these patients typically exhibited hallux limitus, the intraoperative changes of degenerate bone and cartilage uniformly affected greater than 50% of the articular surface of the metatarsal heads, for which the authors provides illustrative evidence (**Fig. 7**). Further, in the majority of these cases there has been a discord between the radiographic classification and the intraoperative findings, suggesting that the clinical and radiographic findings often fall short of the actual degenerative joint disease (**Fig. 6**C compared to **Fig. 7**A illustrates this discord). This finding is supported by a host of articles that fail to correlate severity of the condition with clinical outcome after cheilectomy; the majority of patients respond favorably after this procedure despite the severity of preoperative clinical and radiographic grade or longevity of

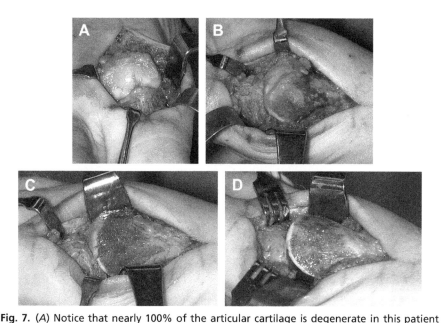

Fig. 7. (*A*) Notice that nearly 100% of the articular cartilage is degenerate in this patient and the metatarsal head appears "bald" without evidence of deep subchondral defects. Plain radiographs revealed the obvious apparent such as the hypertrophic collar of fibrocartilage and joint space narrowing however cannot glean insight as to the true extent of cartilage degeneration in this case. (*B*) Notice the collar of osteophytes and hypertrophic shelf extending over the metatarsal neck. A similar collar of degenerate tissue is found about the phalangeal base giving it an elephant hoof appearance. The medial eminence has an a comma shaped fibrocartilaginous rim which is a thickening of the tubercle for the lateral metatarso-phalangeal ligament. (*C*) With the medial eminence resected and the hypertrophic bone removed from the periphery of the joint a more normal morphology can be appreciated at the joint level. Notice the porous texture and healthy bleeding potential that remains in this metatarsal head which radiographically appeared as a 2nd degree hallux limitus while intraoperatively the metatarsal head was devoid of cartilage. (*D*) Seen here the dorsal 1/3 of the metatarsal head has been resected sparing the central & plantar cartilage and preserving the sesamoid apparatus. Notice the texture of the medial metatarsal head appears much less porous and is comprised of more densely compact bone. A deliberate effort is made to avoid excessive debridement about the interface of the metaphaseal-diaphyseal region as aggressive resection here will lead to post operative capsular adhesions. Notice the base of the phalanx has been debrided to match the contour of the metatarsal head.

symptoms.[8,9,31,39–42,45,47] Further, in this series of patients requiring the modified cheilectomy procedure there was nearly an equal proportion of males and females, which differs from other reports in which females are considered the predominate gender affected by this condition.[8,9,17,21,38,64,65]

Of interest, in 13 of 21 feet there was subtle evidence of medial subluxation at the second MTPJ whereas only 5 of 21 of the second MTPJ's were rectus. This is evidence that the dysfunction of the first MTPJ results in lateral transfer of load, and is the likely culprit for dysfunction with in the second MTPJ complex; specifically the plantar plate. Using the Regnauld classification system for hallux limitus, there were 3 feet graded as first degree, 15 as second degree, and 3 as third degree. Despite the majority of patients being graded as an intermediate degree of bone and joint degeneration (15/21 feet; 71.43%; Regnauld second degree), the intraoperative findings suggested more severe destruction of the joint whereby the patients in this study all seemed to have at least 50% of the articular cartilage defective, if not more. It would seem that osteochondritis of the 1st MTPJ, not unlike that seen in larger joints, evolves insidiously with the radiographic changes lagging behind the clinical progression of the disease. It is understood that 50% to 70% of bone demineralization takes place before radiographic evidence of this bone disease manifests, so the concept of radiographs lagging behind the clinical picture is not a new one. It is

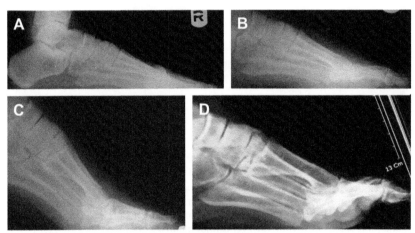

Fig. 8. (A) Seen here the pre operative lateral radiograph depicting the extent of the dorsal osteophyte and joint space narrowing of the 1st MTPJ. The equinated appearance of the hallux is best appreciated in this view. It is easy to appreicate the increased soft tissue density within the soft tissue sleeve of the great toe evidence of the ongoing inflammatory process. (B) This post operative lateral radiograph reveals the conservative extent of bone resection as compared to the pre operative condition noted in (A). (C) Stress lateral radiograph reveals the 1-month post operative range of motion as compared to **Fig. 6**B. It is understood that the morphology of the 1st MTPJ is changed given the bone resection and recontouring. Notice that in the dorsiflexed position there is a plantar hiatus seen at the 1st MTPJ indicative of the liberty about the plantar joint. Should the sesamoid apparatus be fused to the plantar aspect of the joint then this motion would be restricted and no separation of the parts would be visible. It should be noted that there were no adjunctive procedures performed ie, no plantar ligamentous or capsular release. (D) Long term follow up non weight bearing lateral 6-years status post modified cheilectomy there is no evidence of recurrent bone degeneration and the joint contours remain unchanged in comparison with the 1-month post operative lateral view in (B).

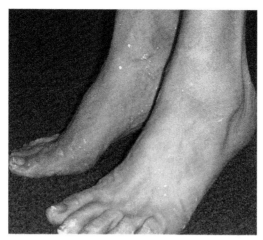

Fig. 9. Clinical evaluation in stance and toe rise reveals non painful joint range of motion with full ability to walk and run at will.

interesting that in this study in 2 of the 3 feet graded as third-degree hallux limitus, stress radiographs revealed preoperative ROM as greater than 40°. After the benefit of the modified cheilectomy, the ROM as documented in the stressed lateral radiographic evaluation was less impressive than the pain reduction reported and the functional outcome; patient's ability to return to earlier activities including kneeling, squatting, and crawling (**Figs. 8** and **9**). This outcome may be explained by the joint decompression reducing peak intra-articular pressures during the propulsive phase of gait while preserving the minimum ROM necessary to propagate through the propulsive phase.[66]

In the 21 feet treated with the modified cheilectomy, the length pattern of the first metatarsal was evaluated and found to be shorter than the second metatarsal in 17 feet, longer than the second metatarsal in 2, and equal to the second metatarsal in 2. In this small group, this does suggest a positive correlation between a short first metatarsal length as compared with the second and hallux limitus. It stands to reason that dysfunction or insufficiency about the first MTPJ would result in lateral transfer of load and stress syndromes within the second ray, which may manifest as second MTPJ instability if not fatigue fracture of the second metatarsal. This concept was further underlined in the current study as 16 of 21 feet demonstrated subtle evidence of 2nd MTPJ subluxation suggesting plantar plate dysfunction coincident with 1st MTPJ insufficiency.

SUMMARY

While there are several theories as to why hallux limitus/rigidus develops, it is clear that painful joint restriction can be alleviated in many cases by the modified cheilectomy. The historical literature reviews a myriad of mechanical influences that may propagate the disease. Foremost, the conditions of medial column dysfunction (often associated with pronatory changes in the rearfoot), metatarsus primus elevatus, and abnormal length patterns of the first metatarsal are considered more than just coincident with the disease. Although these structural and mechanical influences are important, understanding the disease should not be subordinate to such functional discussions. Given the reports of patients requiring surgical intervention for this condition, it is clear that the clinical and radiographic information studied often falls short of the extent of the disease seen in surgery. It is important to understand this discord when developing prognostic information for the patient. To this end it has been realized that the modified cheilectomy has great utility in providing pain relief and improved functional capacity, and in some patients this proves to be a long-standing result. Because the modified cheilectomy has withstood the test of time, it is reasonable to use this method as a first stage in surgical intervention in those patients where the first MTPJ function can and should be restored. Patient selection, taking into consideration functional demand, realistic goals, and the patient's physical well-being, is an integral key to success. It is reasonable to surmise that structural or functional abnormalities, anything that contributes to instability or hypermobility within the first ray will increase the risk of recurrence after even the most meticulous of cheilectomies. Long-term management with the benefit of a prescription orthotic device cannot be understated. While outcomes may vary when considering age groups, athletic activity, and radiographic and clinical grade, there remains an advantage to using the cheilectomy, as it remains a joint-salvage procedure that does not "burn any bridges" sparing as it spares a sufficient foundation of bone should another procedure be required further down the road. The same cannot be said for joint destructive procedures. In fact, given the importance of cost consciousness, if you were to compare these procedures based upon expense the modified cheilectomy is the preferred procedure without debate. The modified cheilectomy has been proven to be an effective, efficient, inexpensive and conservative method that improves 1st MTPJ function with predictable outcomes in appropriate candidates.

REFERENCES

1. Mann RR, Coughlin MJ. Adult hallux valgus. St Louis (MO): Mosby; 1993.
2. Dawson J, Thorogood M, Marks S, et al. The prevalence of foot problems in older women: a cause for concern. J Public Health Med 2002;24:77–84.
3. Menz HB, Lord SR. Gait instability in older people with hallux valgus. Foot Ankle Int 2005;26(61):483–9.
4. Weinfeld SB, Schon L. Hallux metatarsophalangeal arthritis. Clin Orthop Relat Res 1998;249:9–19.
5. vanSaase JL, vanRomunde LK, Cats A, et al. Epidemiology of osteoarthritis: Zoetermeer survey. Comparison of radiological osteoarthritis in a Dutch population with that in 10 other populations. Ann Rheum Dis 1989;48:271–80.
6. Gilheany MF, Landorf KB, Robinson P. Hallux valgus and hallux rigidus: a comparison of impact on health-related quality of life in patients presenting to foot surgeons in Australia. J Foot Ankle Res 2008;1(14):1–6.
7. Feldman R, Hutter J, Lapow L, et al. Cheilectomy and hallux rigidus. J Foot Surg 1983;22:170–4.
8. Feltham G, Hanks S, Marcus R. Age-based outcomes of cheilectomy for the treatment of hallux rigidus. Foot Ankle Int 2001;22:192–7.
9. Mann RA, Coughlin MJ, Duvries HL. Hallux rigidus: a review of the literature and a method of treatment. Clin Orthop 1979;142:57–63.
10. Keogh P, Nagaria J, Stephens M. Cheilectomy for hallux rigidus. Ir J Med Sci 1992;161:681–3.
11. Roukis TS. Review article the need for surgical revision after isolated cheilectomy for hallux rigidus: a systematic review. J Foot Ankle Surg 2010;49:465–70.
12. DuVries H. Static deformities. In: DuVries H, editor. Surgery of the foot. St Louis (MO): Mosby; 1959. p. 392–8.

13. Davies-Colley M. Contraction of the metatarso-phalangeal joint of the great toe. BMJ 1887;1:728.
14. Cotterill J. Stiffness of the great toe in adolescents. BMJ 1888;1:1158.
15. Walsham WJ, Hughes WK. Hallux dolorosus in deformities of the human foot and their treatment. New York: William Wood & Co; 1895. p. 512–4.
16. Goodfellow J. Aetiology of hallux rigidus. Proc R Soc Med 1966;59:821–4.
17. Nilsonne H. Hallux rigidus and its treatment. Acta Orthop Scand 1930;1:295–303.
18. Camasta CA. Hallux limitus and hallux rigidus: clinical examination, radiographic findings, and natural history. Clin Podiatr Med Surg 1996;13:423–47.
19. Lambrinudi P. Metatarsus primus elevatus. Proc R Soc Med 1938;31:1273.
20. Anderson W. Lectures on contractions of the fingers and toes; their varieties, pathology and treatment. Lancet 1891;138:279–82.
21. Bonney G, Macnab I. Hallux valgus and hallux rigidus; a critical survey of operative results. J Bone Joint Surg Br 1952;34(B):366–85.
22. Bingold AC, Collins DH. Hallux rigidus. J Bone Joint Surg Br 1950;32(B):214–22.
23. Shrader JA, Siegel KL. Non operative management of functional hallux limitus in a patient with rheumatoid arthritis. Phys Ther 2003;83:831–43.
24. Jack EA. The aetiology of hallux rigidus. Br J Surg 1940;27:492–7.
25. Cicchinelli LD, Casmasta CA, McGlamry ED. Iatrogenic metatarsus primus elevates. Etiology, evaluation and surgical management. J Am Podiatr Med Assoc 1997;87:165–77.
26. McMurray TP. Treatment of hallux valgus and rigidus. Br Med J 1936;2:218–21.
27. Sim-Fook L, Hodgson AR. A comparison of foot forms among the non-shoe and shoe-wearing Chinese population. J Bone Joint Surg Am 1958;40(A): 1058–62.
28. Grady JF, Axe TM, Zager EJ, et al. A retrospective analysis of 772 patients with hallux limitus. J Am Podiatr Med Assoc 2002;92(2):102–8.
29. Regnauld B. The foot: pathology, aetiology, seminology, clinical investigation and treatment. New York: Springer-Verlag; 1986.
30. Coughlin MJ, Shurnas PS. Hallux rigidus: demographics, etiology and radiographic assessment. Foot Ankle Int 2003;3(24):731–43.
31. Coughlin MJ, Shurnas PS. Treatment of hallux rigidus. Grading and long-term results of operative treatment. J Bone Joint Surg Am 2003;85:2072–88.
32. Coughlin MJ. Conditions of the forefoot. In: DeLee J, Drez D, editors. Orthopaedic sports medicine: principles and practice. Philadelphia: WB Saunders; 1994. p. 221–444.
33. Coughlin MJ, Shurnas PS. Hallux rigidus. J Bone Joint Surg Am 2004; 86(Suppl 1(2)):119–30.
34. Roukis TS, Landsman AS, Ringstrom JB, et al. Distally based capsule periosteum interpositional arthroplasty for hallux rigidus: indications, operative technique and short term follow-up. J Am Podiatr Med Assoc 2003;93(5):349–66.
35. Collier M. Some cases of hallux rigidus; their symptoms, pathology and treatment. Lancet 1894;143(3696):1613–4.
36. McKeever DC. Arthrodesis of the first metatarsophalangeal joint for hallux valgus, hallux rigidus, and metatarsus primus varus. J Bone Joint Surg Am 1952;34: 129–34.
37. Smith NR. Hallux valgus and rigidus treated by arthrodesis of the metatarsophalangeal joint. Br Med J 1952;2:1385–7.
38. Kessel L, Bonney G. Hallux rigidus in the adolescent. J Bone Joint Surg Br 1958; 40(4):668–73.
39. Cochrane WA. An operation for hallux rigidus. Br Med J 1927;1:1095–6.

40. Gould N. Hallux rigidus: cheilotomy or implant? Foot Ankle 1981;1:315.
41. Easley ME, Davis WH, Anderson RB. Intermediate to long-term follow-up of medial-approach dorsal cheilectomy for hallux rigidus. Foot Ankle Int 1999;20:147–52.
42. Geldwert JJ, Rock GD, Mcgrath MP, et al. Cheilectomy: still a useful technique for grade I and grade II hallux limitus/rigidus. J Foot Surg 1992;31:154–9.
43. Mulier T, Steenwerckx A, Thienpont E, et al. Results after cheilectomy in athletes with hallux rigidus. Foot Ankle Int 1999;20:232–7.
44. Hattrup SJ, Johnson KA. Subjective results of hallux rigidus following treatment with cheilectomy. Clin Orthop Relat Res 1988;226:182–91.
45. Lin J, Murphy A. Treatment of hallux rigidus with cheilectomy using a dorsolateral approach. Foot Ankle Int 2009;30:115–9.
46. Thermann H, Becher C, Kilger R. Hallux rigidus treatment with cheilectomy, extensive plantar release, and additional microfracture technique. Tech Foot Ankle Surg 2004;3(4):210–5.
47. Desai VV, Zafiropoulos G, Dias JJ, et al. Hallux rigidus: a case against joint destruction. Presented at the British Orthopaedic Foot Surgery Society Meeting, 12 November 1993. J Bone Joint Surg Br 1994;76(Suppl 2, 3):95.
48. Becher C, Kilger R, Thermann H. Results of cheilectomy and additional microfracture technique for the treatment of hallux rigidus. Foot Ankle Surg 2005;11: 155–60.
49. Coughlin MJ, Shurnas PJ. Soft tissue arthroplasty for hallux rigidus. Foot Ankle Int 2003;24:661–72.
50. Heller WA, Brage ME. The effects of cheilectomy on dorsiflexion of the first metatarsophalangeal joint. Foot Ankle Int 1997;18:803–8.
51. Waizy H, Abbara-Czardybon M, Stukenborg-Colsman C, et al. Mid- and long-term results of the joint preserving therapy of hallux rigidus. Arch Orthop Trauma Surg 2009. Available at: http://www.unboundmedicine.com/medline/ebm/record/ 19306008/full_citation/Mid__and_long_term_results_of_the_joint_preserving_ therapy_of_hallux_rigidus_. Accessed June 23, 2009.
52. Nawoczenski DA, Ketz J, Baumhauer JF. Dynamic kinematic and plantar pressure changes following cheilectomy for hallux rigidus: a mid-term follow-up. Foot Ankle Int 2008;29(3):265–72.
53. Canseco K, Long J, Marks R, et al. Quantitative motion analysis in patients with hallux rigidus before and after cheilectomy. J Orthop Res 2009;27(1): 128–34.
54. Mann RA, Clanton TO. Hallux rigidus: treatment by cheilectomy. J Bone Joint Surg 1988;70A(3):400–6.
55. Mackay DC, Blyth M, Rymaszewski LA. The role of cheilectomy in the treatment of hallux rigidus. J Foot Ankle Surg 1997;36(5):337–40.
56. Shereff MJ, Baumhauer JF. Hallux rigidus and osteoarthritis of the first metatarsophalangeal joint. J Bone Joint Surg Am 1998;80:898–908.
57. Pontell D, Gudas CJ. Retrospective analysis of surgical treatment of hallux rigidus/limitus: clinical and radiographic follow-up of hinged, silastic implant arthroplasty and cheilectomy. J Foot Surg 1988;27:503–10.
58. Lau JT, Daniels TR. Outcomes following cheilectomy and interpositional arthroplasty in hallux rigidus. Foot Ankle Int 2001;22:462–70.
59. Giannestras NJ. Hallux rigidus. In: Foot disorders: medical and surgical management. 2nd edition. Philadelphia: Lea and Febiger; 1973. p. 400–2.
60. Kurtz DH, Harrill JC, Kaczander BI, et al. The Valenti procedure for hallux limitus: a long-term follow-up and analysis. J Foot Ankle Surg 1999;38:123–30.

61. Chang TJ. Stepwise approach to hallux limitus. A surgical perspective. Clin Podiatr Med Surg 1996;13:449–59.
62. Saxena A. The Valenti procedure for hallux limitus/rigidus. J Foot Ankle Surg 1995;34:485–8.
63. Gerbert J. Comment on: "the value of radiographic parameters in the surgical treatment of hallux rigidus" by Zgonis et al, May/June 2005. J Foot Ankle Surg 2005;44(6):494 [author reply: 494].
64. McMaster MJ. The pathogenesis of hallux rigidus. J Bone Joint Surg Br 1978; 60:82.
65. Severin E. Removal of the base of the proximal phalanx for hallux rigidus. Acta Orthop Scand 1947;18:77.
66. Heatherington VJ, Chessman GW, Steuben C. Forces on the 1st metatarsophalangeal joint; A pilot study. J Foot Surg 1992;31(5):450–3.

Multiplanar Phalangeal and Metatarsal Osteotomies for Hallux Rigidus

Brian L. Freeman, DPM[a,b], Mark A. Hardy, DPM[a,c,d],*

KEYWORDS

- Hallux • Rigidus • Limitus • Osteotomy • Operative
- Treatment • Phalangeal • Metatarsal

Hallux limitus was originally described in the literature by Davies-Colley in 1887.[1] Keller claimed the first recorded operative procedure to treat hallux limitus/rigidus in 1904, which involved removal of the base of the proximal phalanx to decompress the arthritic joint. Keller's procedure became the gold standard of operative procedures for many years.[2] In 1938, Lambrinudi[3] described metatarsus primus elevatus, or an elevated first ray, as an entity leading to the formation of hallux limitus owing to dorsal jamming at the first metatarsophalangeal joint (MTPJ). He also described a surgical option aimed at addressing the deformity, with osseous cuts in the metatarsal head that would plantarflex the first metatarsal.

Watermann[4] observed in 1927 that most of the pain with early hallux limitus was at the end range of motion and he described an articular osteotomy to relocate the intact plantar cartilage in a more dorsal position, with a dorsal-based closing wedge osteotomy just behind the articular cartilage of the first metatarsal head.

Bonney and Macnab[5] then described a procedure in 1952 to address some of the lack of motion at the first MTPJ by placing the hallux in a more dorsiflexed attitude relative to the joint with a dorsiflexory base wedge osteotomy of the proximal phalanx. This became the first extra-articular procedure aimed at directly addressing hallux

The authors have nothing to disclose.

[a] Foot and Ankle Residency Program, Cleveland Clinic/Kaiser Permanente, 9500 Euclid Avenue, Cleveland, OH 44195-0002, USA

[b] Department of Orthopedics/Podiatry, Cleveland Clinic Foundation, 9500 Euclid Avenue, Cleveland, OH 44195-0002, USA

[c] Foot and Ankle Trauma Service, Kaiser Permanente–Ohio Region, 10 Severance Circle, Cleveland Heights, Cleveland, OH 44118, USA

[d] Department of Podiatric Surgery, Kaiser Permanente Foundation, 10 Severance Circle, Cleveland Heights, OH 44118, USA

* Corresponding author. Kaiser Permanente Foundation Department of Podiatric Surgery 10 Severance Circle, Cleveland Heights, OH 44118.

E-mail address: markhardy@sbcglobal.net

limitus/rigidus. Around the same time, Mckeever[6] published his article on first MTPJ arthrodesis. Kessel and Bonney[7] later reported on the operative results of the proce-dure in 1958 and the procedure became known as the Bonney-Kessel.

It was not until much later, in 1982, that Youngswick[8] published his article on modi-fications of the Austin bunionectomy that laid the groundwork for many other decompression-type osteotomies that have been proposed and published since that time. This article discusses many of those procedures as well as earlier ones mentioned previously. However, because of the numerous modifications of these procedures and the limited scope of this article, only the most accepted procedures are discussed in detail in this study.

PATHOPHYSIOLOGY OF HALLUX LIMITUS

A number of possible etiologic factors have been proposed for hallux limitus. Root and colleagues[9] identified 7 attributable factors, whereas Lambrinudi had described 4 attrib-utable factors.[3] The possible contributing factors are summarized in **Box 1**. Several investigators have proposed that the primary etiologic factor is previous injury to the joint and that osteochondritis dessicans is the main causative factor, whereas others consider metatarsus primus elevatus to be the primary contributing factor. More recently it has been shown that an elongated hallux can lead to the formation of hallux rigidus.[10,11] For a more thorough discussion on this topic, please read Dr Botek's article elsewhere in this issue on "Etiology, Pathophysiology and Staging of Hallux Rigidus."

PHALANGEAL OSTEOTOMIES IN THE TREATMENT OF HALLUX RIGIDUS
Keller and Interpositional Arthroplasty

First described by Davies-Colley[1] in 1887 and later popularized by Keller[2] in 1904, the Keller[21] arthroplasty has been one of the mainstays of the treatment of hallux rigidus (**Fig. 1**). It consists of removing the base of the proximal phalanx and releasing its respective soft tissue attachments as well as removing the medial eminence of the first metatarsal head, which is often combined with exostectomy of the metatarsal head. It is indicated in severe/end-stage hallux rigidus, particularly in the elderly population, or iatrogenic hallux rigidus, making it unique in relation to the other osteotomies dis-cussed in this article, which are indicated in younger, active populations with mild

---

Box 1
Factors attributing to hallux limitus/rigidus

1. Paralytic deformities[3]
2. Severe pes planovalgus[12,13]
3. Long first metatarsal[5,14]
4. Hypermobility of the first ray[9]
5. Metatarsus primus elevatus[3,7,9,12]
6. Ankylosis secondary to gout, psoriatic arthritis, rheumatoid arthritis[9,15]
7. Trauma[9,16]
8. Osteochondritis dessicans[16–18]
9. Iatrogenic[12,19]
10. Flat or chevron-shaped metatarsal head[10]
11. Long phalanx[10,11,20]

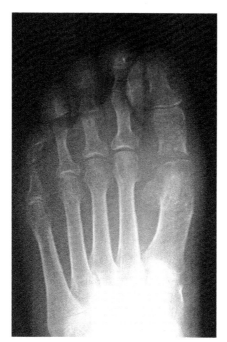

Fig. 1. Keller procedure.

to moderate hallux limitus/rigidus. It requires no bone healing and is therefore indicated in patients with poor bone-healing potential with low functional demands and who may be unable to remain non–weight bearing after surgery to heal a more aggressive procedure, such as a first MTPJ arthrodesis.[22] Some of the complications involved with the procedure include cock-up deformity of the hallux, transfer lesions, loss of power with toe-off, and flail hallux. Although some of the complications can be avoided by correct surgical technique, it is inherently an unstable procedure that has a mind of its own and, according to Lau and Daniels,[23] should be considered a salvage procedure because of its unpredictability.

Initially there was no interposition of soft tissue following the resection of the phalangeal base and practically no fixation. Later, many found that interpositional soft tissue grafts of varying sources helped maintain motion in the joint, provided less postoperative pain, and provided potential extended functionality of the first ray either by preserving some of its length or by reattaching some soft tissue structures to the interposed graft.[19,22–30] Schenk and colleagues[31] argued that this was not the case, and in a study of 52 feet found no difference between patients treated with the traditional Keller and those treated with interposition arthroplasty. The use of Kirschner wire (K-wire) fixation crossing the first MTPJ has been advocated by Vallier and colleagues[32–34] to maintain a better position of the hallux postoperatively and to reduce metatarsalgia, but results have varied on this topic.

The question of how much of the proximal phalanx should be resected has been addressed by numerous investigators and studies. The overall consensus seems to be to resect enough, but not too much, and to limit resection to about 33%.[32,35] Limiting resection lessens the occurrence of a cock-up deformity of the hallux and maintains more load-bearing potential by the hallux.[35–37] Quinn and colleagues[38] tried to address this shortening with a procedure similar to that of Regnauld by removing the base, remodeling it, shortening it, and then reinserting it. They obtained good over-all results in their small study group, but the procedure retained the same shortfalls as the original Regnauld and has not gained popularity.

Another use of the Keller has been in hallux abducto valgus (HAV) surgery, and some promote it as a viable option in elderly individuals with low functional demand and/or poor bone-healing potential, reporting that it could reduce the intermetatarsal and metatarsophalangeal angles as well as reduce pain at the first MTPJ.[32,39–42] Its use has been discouraged in patients with severe HAV, as the effect on the intermetatarsal angle is minor. It has also been promoted for treatment of nonhealing interphalangeal joint (IPJ) ulcerations in the neuropathic patient, but research to support its use and long-term complications, such as transfer lesions and ulcers, have not been followed adequately.[43,44]

Kessel-Bonney

The Kessel-Bonney procedure is a dorsiflexory wedge osteotomy of the proximal phalanx of the hallux (**Fig. 2**). Its purpose is not to allow more joint motion but to cause a more dorsiflexed hallux relative to the first MTPJ, thus allowing more functional dorsiflexion of the hallux during gait.

Bonney and Macnab[5] first proposed the procedure in 1952 as they were exploring osteotomies in the treatment of hallux rigidus for adolescent patients after experiencing very poor results with a Keller arthroplasty in a young female patient. The results and short-term outcomes of their procedure were later reported in 1958 by Kessel and Bonney[7] with relatively good results.

The Kessel-Bonney procedure was initially intended only for adolescent patients 18 years or younger with minimal to no joint disease apparent on radiographs; however, more recently it has been used on older patients with mild to moderate hallux rigidus.[45–47] The primary indication still remains limited dorsiflexion with adequate plantarflexion at the first MTPJ with minimal to no degenerative changes or osteophyte formation. It is not recommended in the elderly or in patients with poor bone-healing potential, or in those with severe disease (stage 3).

There are several benefits of the Kessel-Bonney procedure, which include maintenance of the metatarsal parabola, avoidance of violating the first MTPJ capsule, and a relatively stable osteotomy if the plantar cortex is left intact. The ability to increase the perceived range of motion without modifying the metatarsal parabola is one of

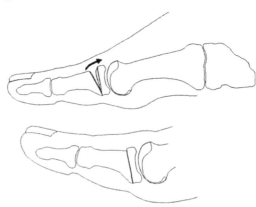

Fig. 2. Bonney-Kessel procedure. (*From* Muscarella V, Hetherington VJ. Hallux limitus and hallux rigidus. In: Hetherington VJ, editor. New York: Churchill Livingstone; 1994. p. 323; with permission.)

the major benefits of this procedure. Whereas metatarsal osteotomies often strive to decompress and plantarflex the first MTPJ to maintain its contact with the ground and to avoid excess loading of the lateral metatarsals, the Kessel-Bonney procedure avoids this complication by maintaining the parabola and allowing the intrinsic musculature on the base of the proximal phalanx to remain intact, thus lessening the incidence of transfer pain or lesions (**Table 1**).[47,48]

As the procedure includes the cutting and healing of bone, there are a number of possible adverse effects. One of the major complications includes the possibility of injuring the growing physis in adolescent patients, which must be carefully avoided with preoperative and intraoperative planning.[49] One of the best long-term follow-ups for the procedure comes from Citron and Neil,[50] who reported in 1987 on 10 procedures in 8 female patients (ages 10 to 52) who they followed for an average of 22 years. Their complications included secondary osteoarthrosis of the IPJ of the hallux because of compensatory plantarflexion in one patient, which required an IPJ fusion; a malunion in another case; and a painful nonunion in one patient that necessitated fusion of the first MTPJ. Nine of the 10 procedures demonstrated diminished joint space at the first MTPJ when compared with initial radiographs.

In 2005, Kilmartin followed a group of 49 patients undergoing phalangeal osteotomy over an average of 29 months. Of those, 65% were completely satisfied, 24% were moderately satisfied, and 11% were dissatisfied. Complications included metatarsalgia (8%), continued first MTPJ pain (7%), IPJ joint pain (6%), delayed union (4%), and internal fixation that necessitated removal (8%) (see **Box 1**). Kilmartin[47] also compared his findings to patients undergoing metatarsal decompression osteotomies.

More recently, there have been several studies that have produced very good results when the Kessel-Bonney was used as an adjunctive procedure in combination with a cheilectomy or decompression osteotomy. These studies recommended cheilectomy with a dorsiflexory osteotomy as first-line treatment for stage 1 and 2 hallux rigidus, especially for those with continued limited range of motion at the first MTPJ after a cheilectomy has been performed.[45,48,51,52]

Regnauld

In 1986, Regnauld[53] described an enclavement procedure, a "peg-in-hole" technique. It consisted of removing the base of the proximal phalanx and resecting a cylinder of

Table 1
Phalangeal osteotomy and first metatarsal decompression osteotomy complications

Complication	Phalangeal Osteotomy, n = 49 (%)	First Metatarsal Osteotomy, n = 59 (%)
Metatarsalgia	4(8)	18(30)
Stress fracture, 2nd metatarsal	0	4(7)
Continued first MTPJ pain	3(7)	2(3)
Hallux IPJ pain	3(6)	0
Delayed union	2(4)	3(5)
Avascular necrosis	0	2(3)
Infection	0	1(2)
Internal fixation removal	4(8)	8(13)

Abbreviations: IPJ, interphalangeal joint; MTPJ, metatarsophalangeal joint.
Data from Kilmartin TE. Phalangeal osteotomy versus first metatarsal decompression osteotomy for the surgical treatment of hallux rigidus: a prospective study of age-matched and condition-matched patients. J Foot Ankle Surg 2005;44(1):2–12.

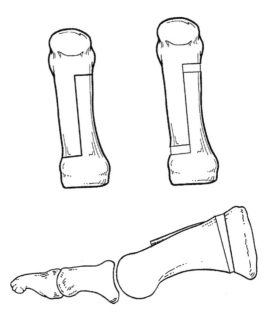

Fig. 3. Sagittal Z procedure.

bone. The remaining exposed end of the proximal phalanx was then reduced so that the base with the removed cylinder would fit snugly on the proximal phalanx, and the two were then pieced together. Regnauld initially described 3 graft shapes: hat, cork, and inverted. The reason for the procedure was to remove about one-third of the proximal phalanx so as to decompress the joint. In 1992, Cohen[54] implemented screw fixation of the graft that avoided some of the complications present with the original unfixed method. Quinn and collegues[38] also reported on the procedure, calling it a modified Keller. Among the positive benefits discovered were early range of motion, no implanted materials, preservation of articular surfaces, and the option of revisional surgeries. The most notable complication includes resorption of the graft owing to the devascularization caused by graft removal. Despite the reported initial success with the procedure, it failed to gain much popularity, most likely because it was technically demanding and time consuming to perform.

Sagittal "Z"

Although never described alone, the sagittal Z osteotomy described by Kissel and colleagues[55] offered good results when combined with aggressive cheilectomy and chondroplasty at the first MTPJ (**Fig. 3**). However, it does not offer significant benefit in functional outcome when compared with the traditional Kessel-Bonney procedure, and was recommended only in the young active patient; hence, it has not been thoroughly studied. The 2 major advantages of the sagittal Z include greater ability to fixate with a screw and greater shortening potential versus the Kessel-Bonney, while avoiding the avascular necrosis and excessive dissection associated with the Regnauld procedure.[56]

DISTAL METATARSAL OSTEOTOMIES IN THE TREATMENT OF HALLUX RIGIDUS
Weil/Mau/Distal Oblique Osteotomy

The distal oblique osteotomy (Weil) is most closely associated with lesser metatarsalgia to decompress a joint and reduce the length of a metatarsal, and has similar

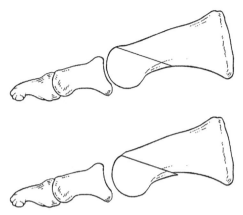

Fig. 4. Weil/Mau/Distal oblique osteotomy.

indications in the treatment of hallux limitus (**Fig. 4**). It can also be used to shorten a long metatarsal, plantarflex an elevated metatarsal, decompress a painful joint, and to address a mild increase in the first intermetatarsal angle. It is a transverse plane osteotomy angled from dorsal distal to plantar proximal with the angle of the cut ranging from 35 to 45 degrees.[57] Ronconi and colleagues[57] studied 26 patients on whom both the Weil and an aggressive cheilectomy were performed, with 84% having good to excellent results.

LaMar and colleagues[58] performed a mechanical comparison on bone models of the Youngswick, sagittal V, and modified Weil osteotomies. Each osteotomy was fixated with one screw. They found no statistically significant difference in strength between the Youngswick and Weil, but did find that the sagittal V was drastically weaker than the previous two.

The reason some would use the Weil rather than another decompression osteotomy is because of its versatility. It is a 1-cut osteotomy versus the 2 to 5 cuts needed for many of the other procedures. With it, the surgeon is able to plantarflex and shorten, although the degree to which each of these separate objectives is accomplished depends on the degree at which the cut is made. A more vertical cut allows more plantarflexion and less shortening, whereas a more horizontal cut permits more shortening and less plantarflexion. If fixated with 2 screws, as performed by Ronconi and colleagues,[57] it offers a very stable construct as well. More studies are needed to determine its effectiveness and strength in vivo compared with the other distal metatarsal osteotomies in the treatment of hallux limitus.

Youngswick

Since first described in 1982, the Youngswick has become one of the most popular distal metatarsal osteotomies used in hallux rigidus treatment. Its main indications include an elevated metatarsal head and/or long first metatarsal in the presence of hallux limitus with or without concomitant hallux abductovalgus. It has also been proposed that by plantarflexing and shortening the metatarsal head, this procedure can be used to increase joint mobility and reduce pain in patients with hallux limitus without the previously named indications by decreasing resistance between the metatarsal head and the sesamoids during weight bearing.[59]

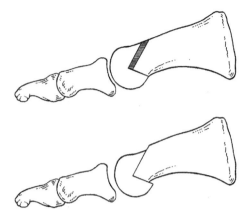

Fig. 5. Youngswick procedure.

It is essentially a modified Austin procedure with a 60-degree angled cut in which a section of bone is removed from the dorsal arm of the osteotomy (**Fig. 5**).[8] When the section of bone is removed, the metatarsal head slides posteriorly and plantarly. If the angle of the cuts is varied and the plantar arm becomes more parallel with the weight-bearing surface, it is possible to obtain shortening of the head with minimal to no plantarflexion.[60] Fixation is similar to the Austin bunionectomy and offers the advantage of being inherently stable in all 3 cardinal planes when 1 point of fixation is used. If the patient has an increased intermetatarsal angle along with an elongated first metatarsal, both may be addressed concomitantly with the Youngswick procedure.[61]

As it is somewhat difficult to plantarflex without shortening with the traditional Youngswick procedure, Radovic and colleagues[62] recently described a modification that allows minimal shortening with a greater ability to plantarflex by taking the section of bone removed from the dorsal arm and inserting it into the plantar arm as an autogenous graft.

Watermann

The original Watermann[4] consisted of the removal of a dorsally based trapezoidal wedge from the first metatarsal head. Its purpose was to relocate the viable plantar cartilage to a more dorsal location relative to the proximal phalanx, thus allowing more dorsiflexion of the hallux (**Fig. 6**). Besides relocating the cartilage, it also decompressed the joint by reducing its internal cubic content, thereby relaxing the surrounding soft tissue structures and allowing more joint motion.[63] It is generally indicated in younger active patients with minimal to no degeneration of the first MTPJ when decompression is sought to relieve joint pain. It has also been used in conjunction with a proximal plantarflexory osteotomy for treatment of metatarsus elevatus, described by Drago and colleagues[64] and Cavolo and colleagues.[63]

The Watermann procedure is inherently unstable, as the bone cut is perpendicular to the shaft of the bone and does not offer easy fixation especially because of its close proximity to the joint. It also provides little of the structural stability of the Youngswick procedure. Care must be taken when performing the procedure to avoid damaging the sesamoid apparatus directly below the osteotomy. It is contraindicated in metatarsus primus elevatus, as it may exacerbate the disorder.[65]

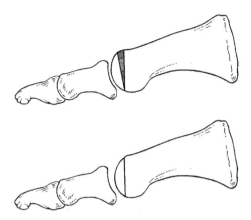

Fig. 6. Watermann procedure.

Watermann Green

The name Watermann Green is somewhat misleading, as it does not offer rotation of the articular cartilage like the original Watermann, and must therefore be considered an entirely unique procedure. It was devised after it became apparent that the Watermann alone was inadequate to fully decompress the joint and to address the dorsal exostosis in more progressed hallux limitus.[66] The Watermann Green involves a 2-arm osteotomy in the metatarsal head, with the dorsal arm being parallel to the long axis of the bone and the plantar arm being parallel to the weight-bearing surface. A dorsal cheilectomy is frequently performed in conjunction with the procedure (**Fig. 7**). A dorsal section of bone is removed, allowing for shortening and decompression of the first MTPJ, as well as correction of the proximal articular set angle (PASA), if existent, when a trapezoidal section is removed. It is also possible to mildly plantarflex the head if the plantar arm is angled more plantarly versus being parallel to the weight-bearing surface.[67]

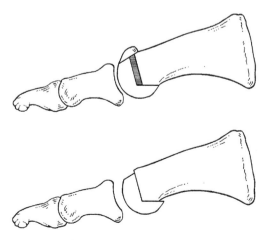

Fig. 7. Green-Watermann procedure.

The advantages of the Watermann Green over the original Watermann include the following:

1. Avoidance of the sesamoid apparatus
2. More stable osteotomy with greater ease of fixation
3. Greater decompression
4. Correction of the PASA of the first MTPJ
5. Plantarflexion of the metatarsal head.

The main disadvantage is the inability to rotate the viable plantar articular cartilage in a more dorsal attitude. Dickerson and colleagues[68] reported on 32 patients who underwent the procedure on 40 toes, with an average follow-up of 4 years, with 94% stating that the procedure had greatly reduced their first MTPJ pain. In comparison with the Youngswick procedure, the Watermann Green is less stable, with the main advantage of the latter being the ability to adjust for the PASA at the first MTPJ.

Tricorrectional Osteotomy

Initially proposed as a treatment method for bunions, the tricorrectional distal metatarsal osteotomy has shown some positive results in the treatment of end-stage hallux rigidus, according to Selner and colleagues.[69–74] The procedure is similar to the Youngswick and Watermann Green procedures, but with more adjustment of the axis guide to allow greater shortening if the patient has a concomitant HAV deformity or the removal of a trapezoidal piece of bone if it is desired to adjust for PASA. Selner and colleagues[69] accomplished good results in 17 of 19 patients treated with severe joint disease and severely decreased range of motion at the first MTPJ. The reason this procedure can be used in severe hallux limitus, while the Youngswick and Watermann Green cannot, has yet to be addressed. It is a technically demanding procedure to perform, but is easy to fixate with one cortical screw placement similar to an Austin procedure.

Mayo-Stone

The Mayo-Stone procedure is of historical importance only. It consisted of an angled cut, usually around 45 degrees from dorsal proximal to plantar distal to the plantar joint space of the first MTPJ. In the past 30 years, very little has been written about the procedure, although its cousin the Valenti procedure, which involves a similar cut on the metatarsal head and the reverse on the proximal phalangeal base, is still in use. Please see Dr Judge's article elsewhere in this issue on "First Metatarsophalangeal Joint Cheilectomy and its Modifications" for further discussion on the Valenti procedure. The procedure's intent was to produce a similar affect to the Keller without sacrificing the soft tissue attachments on the plantar surface of the joint.

Sagittal V and the Long-Arm Decompression Osteotomy

The sagittal V is not well studied, for its construct was shown to be weak in comparison with other plantarflexory decompression distal osteotomies of the first metatarsal.[58] A long-arm modification of it, termed the long-arm decompression osteotomy (LADO), was proposed by Robinson and Frank[75] as an intermediate to the distal decompression osteotomies and the more proximal plantarflexory osteotomies. They reported that it offered the possibility of greater shortening and greater plantarflexion than its more distal counterparts, while being more stable than the proximal osteotomies, as well as presenting less likelihood of troughing than the sagittal Z osteotomy, while still retaining the possibility of 2-screw fixation. In 2005, when

Robinson and Frank[75] published their hypothesis, they had performed the procedure on only 2 patients and have yet to report on further outcomes.

PROXIMAL METATARSAL OSTEOTOMIES IN THE TREATMENT OF HALLUX RIGIDUS
Plantarflexory Closing Base Wedge/Lambrinudi

Lambrinudi[3] introduced his procedure in 1938, addressing what he termed "metatarsus primus elevatus." It is indicated in patients with metatarsus primus elevatus with minimal to no shortening of the first metatarsal needed in stage 0–1 hallux limitus. Davies[76] later reported on the procedure as something to consider in the correct patient population, noting that it may slow or change the progression of degenerative joint disease at the first MTPJ while observing that it took considerably more time for a patient to heal from the procedure when compared with other forefoot procedures. One of the disadvantages of the procedure includes the need to be very precise in the amount of bone resected so as not to plantarflex the metatarsal head excessively, whereas the sagittal Z offers a correction that can be adjusted more readily.

Sagittal Z/Sagittal Scarf

Proximal metatarsal osteotomies in the treatment of hallux limitus offer several advantages over distal metatarsal osteotomies. First, they can be used to plantarflex more aggressively. Second, they can provide plantarflexion without shortening and often allow the surgeon to dial in correction more precisely. Third, they facilitate elongation of a metatarsal if needed. Because they deal with cortical instead of cancellous bone, they do incur the risk of troughing and delayed healing and often require the patient to be non–weight bearing for a period of time.[77]

The sagittal Z is performed with the distal arm exiting laterally and the proximal arm exiting medially, with the central arm running the length of the diaphysis, perpendicular to the weight-bearing surface. When shortening is required, a section of bone is removed from both the distal and proximal arms. After the osteotomies are performed, the distal aspect of the metatarsal can then be rotated to accomplish the desired plantarflexion.[77]

Many investigators have reported on the good outcomes of the procedure. Cicchinelli and colleagues[19] recommended it as the procedure of choice in patients with metatarsus primus elevatus with attendant hallux limitus. Viegas[78] followed 11 patients who had the procedure with good to excellent results in all of them. At a 2-year follow-up, Chang[79] reported 86% good results on 32 cases, and found the sagittal Z to be the most versatile of the proximal metatarsal osteotomies for hallux limitus.

Drago

The Drago osteotomy is a double osteotomy consisting of an opening plantarflexory base wedge osteotomy in conjunction with a Watermann procedure (**Fig. 8**). The base wedge was performed by taking the bone removed from the Watermann procedure distally and using it as the distracting graft for the base osteotomy. Drago and colleagues'[64] reasoning for the double osteotomy was the idea that plantarflexing the metatarsal would cause the articular surface to take on a more plantarflexed attitude, thereby adding to the dorsal jamming at the joint. The Watermann was then performed to counteract the jamming produced, thus allowing more plantarflexion of the first metatarsal in comparison with the more distally based osteotomies.[64]

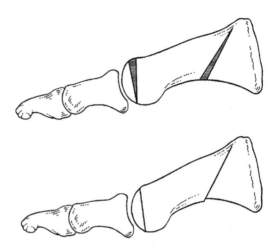

Fig. 8. Drago procedure.

SUMMARY

As one can see, there are a variety of joint-salvaging procedures available for treatment of hallux limitus/rigidus. Each of the procedures discussed in this article provides a very viable alternative to arthrodesis. Procedure selection depends on a number of factors. These include, but are not limited to, ambulatory status, concomitant hallux valgus or multiplane deformity, sesamoid arthrosis, metatarsal parabola, lesser metatarsalgia, and medical comorbidities. The advantages and disadvantages of each procedure need to be weighed with the expectations of both the surgeon and the patient.

REFERENCES

1. Davies-Colley N. Contraction of the metatarsophalangeal joint of the great toe (hallux flexus). Br Med J 1887;1:728.
2. Keller WL. The surgical treatment of bunions and hallux valgus. NY Med J 1904; 80:741–2.
3. Lambrinudi C. Metatarsus primus elevatus. Proc R Soc Med 1938;31(11):1273.
4. Watermann H. Die arthritis deformans grosszehengrundge-lenkes. Orthop Chir 1927;48:346–55.
5. Bonney G, Macnab I. Hallux valgus and hallux rigidus: a critical survey of operative results. J Bone Joint Surg Br 1952;34(3):366–85.
6. Mckeever DC. Arthrodesis of the first metatarsophalangeal joint for hallux valgus, hallux rigidus, and metatarsus primus varus. J Bone Joint Surg Am 1952;34(1): 129–34.
7. Kessel L, Bonney G. Hallux rigidus in the adolescent. J Bone Joint Surg Br 1958; 40(4):668–73.
8. Youngswick FD. Modifications of the Austin bunionectomy for treatment of metatarsus primus elevatus associated with hallux limitus. J Foot Surg 1982;21(2): 114–6.
9. Root ML, Orien WP, Weed JH. Normal and abnormal function of the foot. Los Angeles (CA): Clinical Biomechanics Corporation; 1977. p. 358–62.

10. Beeson P, Phillips C, Corr S, et al. Cross-sectional study to evaluate radiological parameters in hallux rigidus. Foot (Edinb) 2009;19(1):7–21.
11. Zammit GV, Menz HB, Munteanu SE. Structural factors associated with hallux limitus/rigidus: a systematic review of case control studies. J Orthop Sports Phys Ther 2009;39(10):733–42.
12. Meyer JO, Nishon LR, Weiss L, et al. Metatarsus primus elevatus and the etiology of hallux rigidus. J Foot Surg 1987;26(3):237–41.
13. Jansen M. Hallux valgus, rigidus and malleus. J Bone Joint Surg 1921;3(3):87.
14. Nilsonne H. Hallux rigidus and its treatment. Acta Orthop Scand 1930;1(1–4):295.
15. Karasick D, Wapner KL. Hallux rigidus deformity: radiologic assessment. AJR Am J Roentgenol 1991;157(5):1029–33.
16. Goodfellow J. Aetiology of hallux rigidus. Proc R Soc Med 1966;59(9):821–4.
17. McMaster MJ. The pathogenesis of hallux rigidus. J Bone Joint Surg Br 1978; 60(1):82–7.
18. Vilaseca RR, Ribes ER. The growth of the first metatarsal bone. Foot Ankle 1980; 1(2):117–22.
19. Cicchinelli LD, Camasta CA, McGlamry ED. Iatrogenic metatarsus primus elevatus. Etiology, evaluation, and surgical management. J Am Podiatr Med Assoc 1997;87(4):165–77.
20. Munuera PV, Dominguez G, Castillo JM. Radiographic study of the size of the first metatarso-digital segment in feet with incipient hallux limitus. J Am Podiatr Med Assoc 2007;97(6):460–8.
21. Keller WL. Further observations on the surgical treatment of hallux valgus and bunions. NY Med J 1912;88(4):696–9.
22. Brage ME, Ball ST. Surgical options for salvage of end-stage hallux rigidus. Foot Ankle Clin 2002;7(1):49–73.
23. Lau JT, Daniels TR. Outcomes following cheilectomy and interpositional arthroplasty in hallux rigidus. Foot Ankle Int 2001;22(6):462–70.
24. Hahn MP, Gerhardt N, Thordarson DB. Medial capsular interpositional arthroplasty for severe hallux rigidus. Foot Ankle Int 2009;30(6):494–9.
25. Becerro de Bengoa Vallejo R, Losa Iglesias ME, Viejo Tirado F, et al. Use of a Kirschner wire for distraction and capsular flaps in the Keller interpositional arthroplasty. J Am Podiatr Med Assoc 2008;98(4):326–9.
26. Berlet GC, Hyer CF, Lee TH, et al. Interpositional arthroplasty of the first MTP joint using a regenerative tissue matrix for the treatment of advanced hallux rigidus. Foot Ankle Int 2008;29(1):10–21.
27. Roukis TS, Landsman AS, Ringstrom JB, et al. Distally based capsule-periosteum interpositional arthroplasty for hallux rigidus. Indications, operative technique, and short-term follow-up. J Am Podiatr Med Assoc 2003;93(5):349–66.
28. Cosentino GL. The Cosentino modification for tendon interpositional arthroplasty. J Foot Ankle Surg 1995;34(5):501–8.
29. Kolker D, Weinfeld S. Technique tip: a modification to the Keller arthroplasty using interposition allograft. Foot Ankle Int 2007;28(2):266–8.
30. Mroczek KJ, Miller SD. The modified oblique Keller procedure: a technique for dorsal approach interposition arthroplasty sparing the flexor tendons. Foot Ankle Int 2003;24(7):521–2.
31. Schenk S, Meizer R, Kramer R, et al. Resection arthroplasty with and without capsular interposition for treatment of severe hallux rigidus. Int Orthop 2009; 33(1):145–50.
32. Vallier GT, Petersen SA, LaGrone MO. The Keller resection arthroplasty: a 13-year experience. Foot Ankle 1991;11(4):187–94.

33. McLaughlin EK, Fish C. Keller arthroplasty: is distraction a useful technique? A retrospective study. J Foot Surg 1990;29(3):223–5.

34. Sherman KP, Douglas DL, Benson MK. Keller's arthroplasty: is distraction useful? A prospective trial. J Bone Joint Surg Br 1984;66(5):765–9.

35. Breitenseher MJ, Toma CD, Gottsauner-Wolf F, et al. Hallux rigidus operated on by Keller and Brandes method: radiological parameters of success and prognosis. Rofo 1996;164(6):483–8.

36. Love TR, Whynot AS, Farine I, et al. Keller arthroplasty: a prospective review. Foot Ankle 1987;8(1):46–54.

37. Henry AP, Waugh W, Wood H. The use of footprints in assessing the results of operations for hallux valgus. A comparison of Keller's operation and arthrodesis. J Bone Joint Surg Br 1975;57(4):478–81.

38. Quinn M, Wolf K, Hensley J, et al. Keller arthroplasty with autogenous bone graft in the treatment of hallux limitus. J Foot Surg 1990;29(3):284–91.

39. Donley BG, Vaughn RA, Stephenson KA, et al. Keller resection arthroplasty for treatment of hallux valgus deformity: increased correction with fibular sesamoidectomy. Foot Ankle Int 2002;23(8):699–703.

40. Kissel CG, Mistretta RP, Morse RL. Reduction of intermetatarsal angle following Keller arthroplasty. J Foot Ankle Surg 1993;32(2):193–6.

41. Kitaoka HB, Patzer GL. Arthrodesis versus resection arthroplasty for failed hallux valgus operations. Clin Orthop Relat Res 1998;(347):208–14.

42. Schneider W, Knahr K. Keller procedure and chevron osteotomy in hallux valgus: five-year results of different surgical philosophies in comparable collectives. Foot Ankle Int 2002;23(4):321–9.

43. Dannels E. Neuropathic foot ulcer prevention in diabetic American Indians with hallux limitus. J Am Podiatr Med Assoc 1989;79(9):447–50.

44. Stewart J, Reed JF 3rd. An audit of Keller arthroplasty and metatarsophalangeal joint arthrodesis from national data. Int J Low Extrem Wounds 2003;2(2):69–73.

45. Waizy H, Czardybon MA, Stukenborg-Colsman C, et al. Mid- and long-term results of the joint preserving therapy of hallux rigidus. Arch Orthop Trauma Surg 2010;130(2):165–70.

46. Moberg E. A simple operation for hallux rigidus. Clin Orthop Relat Res 1979;(142): 55–6.

47. Kilmartin TE. Phalangeal osteotomy versus first metatarsal decompression osteotomy for the surgical treatment of hallux rigidus: a prospective study of age-matched and condition-matched patients. J Foot Ankle Surg 2005;44(1):2–12.

48. Thomas PJ, Smith RW. Proximal phalanx osteotomy for the surgical treatment of hallux rigidus. Foot Ankle Int 1999;20(1):3–12.

49. Coughlin MJ, Mann RA. Surgery of the foot and ankle. St Louis (MO): Mosby; 1999. p. 615.

50. Citron N, Neil M. Dorsal wedge osteotomy of the proximal phalanx for hallux rigidus. Long-term results. J Bone Joint Surg Br 1987;69(5):835–7.

51. Roukis TS. Outcomes after cheilectomy with phalangeal dorsiflexory osteotomy for hallux rigidus: a systematic review. J Foot Ankle Surg 2010;45(5):479–87.

52. Makwana NK. Osteotomy of the hallux proximal phalanx. Foot Ankle Clin 2001; 6(3):455–71.

53. Regnauld B. In: Elson R, editor. The foot: pathology, aetiology, semiology, clinical investigation and therapy. Berlin: Springer-Verlag; 1986. p. 335–50.

54. Cohen M, Roman A, Liessner P. A modification of the Regnauld procedure for hallux limitus. J Foot Surg 1992;31(5):498–503.

55. Kissel CG, Mistretta RP, Unroe BJ. Cheilectomy, chondroplasty, and sagittal "Z" osteotomy: a preliminary report on an alternative joint preservation approach to hallux limitus. J Foot Ankle Surg 1995;34(3):312–8.
56. Hodor L, Hess T. Shortening Z-osteotomy for the proximal phalanx of the hallux using axial guides. J Am Podiatr Med Assoc 1995;85(5):249–54.
57. Ronconi P, Monachino P, Baleanu PM, et al. Distal oblique osteotomy of the first metatarsal for the correction of hallux limitus and rigidus deformity. J Foot Ankle Surg 2000;39(3):154–60.
58. LaMar L, Deroy AR, Sinnot MT, et al. Mechanical comparison of the Youngswick, sagittal V, and modified Weil osteotomies for hallux rigidus in a sawbone model. J Foot Ankle Surg 2006;45(2):70–5.
59. Bryant AR, Tinley P, Cole JH. Plantar pressure and joint motion after the Youngswick procedure for hallux limitus. J Am Podiatr Med Assoc 2004;94(1):22–30.
60. Gerbert J, Moadab A, Rupley KF. Youngswick-Austin procedure: the effect of plantar arm orientation on metatarsal head displacement. J Foot Ankle Surg 2001;40(1):8–14.
61. Boberg J, Ruch JA, Banks AS. Distal metaphyseal osteotomies in hallux abducto valgus surgery. In: McGlamry ED, editor. Comprehensive textbook of foot surgery. Baltimore (MD): Williams & Wilkins; 1987. p. 173–84.
62. Radovic P, Yadav-Shah E, Choe K. Modified Youngswick procedure for hallux limitus. J Am Podiatr Med Assoc 2007;97(5):420–3.
63. Cavolo DJ, Cavallaro DC, Arrington LE. The Watermann osteotomy for hallux limitus. J Am Podiatry Assoc 1979;69(1):52–7.
64. Drago JJ, Oloff L, Jacobs AM. A comprehensive review of hallux limitus. J Foot Surg 1984;23(3):213–20.
65. Beeson P. The surgical treatment of hallux limitus/rigidus: a critical review of the literature. Foot 2009;14(1):6–22.
66. Laakman G, Green R, Green DR. The modified Watermann procedure a preliminary retrospective study. In: Camasta CA, editor. Reconstructive surgery of the foot and leg update. Tucker (GA): The Podiatry Institute; 1995. p. 128–35.
67. Feldman KA. The Green-Watermann procedure: geometric analysis and preoperative radiographic template technique. J Foot Surg 1992;31(2):182–5.
68. Dickerson JB, Green R, Green DR. Long-term follow-up of the Green-Watermann osteotomy for hallux limitus. J Am Podiatr Med Assoc 2002;92(10):543–54.
69. Selner AJ, Bogdan R, Selner MD, et al. Tricorrectional osteotomy for the correction of late-stage hallux limitus/rigidus. J Am Podiatr Med Assoc 1997;87(9):414–24.
70. Boggs SI, Selner AJ, Roth IE, et al. Tricorrectional bunionectomy with AO screw fixation. J Foot Surg 1989;28(3):185–90.
71. Selner AJ, Selner MD, Tucker RA, et al. Tricorrectional bunionectomy for surgical repair of juvenile hallux valgus. J Am Podiatr Med Assoc 1992;82(1):21–4.
72. Selner AJ, Ginex SL, Selner MD. Tricorrectional bunionectomy for correction of high intermetatarsal angles. J Am Podiatr Med Assoc 1994;84(8):385–9.
73. Selner AJ, King SA, Samuels DI, et al. Tricorrectional bunionectomy for hallux abducto valgus. A comprehensive outcome study. J Am Podiatr Med Assoc 1999;89(4):174–82.
74. Selner AJ, Selner MD, Cyr RP, et al. Revisional hallux abducto valgus surgery using tricorrectional bunionectomy. J Am Podiatr Med Assoc 2004;94(4):341–6.
75. Robinson SC, Frank RP. Long arm decompression osteotomy for hallux limitus. Clin Podiatr Med Surg 2005;22(2):301–7, vii.
76. Davies GF. Plantarflexory base wedge osteotomy in the treatment of functional and structural metatarsus primus elevatus. Clin Podiatr Med Surg 1989;6(1):93–102.

77. Chang TJ, Camasta CA. Hallux limitus and hallus rigidus. In: Banks AS, Downey MS, editors. McGlamry's comprehensive textbook of foot and ankle surgery. Lippincott Williams & Wilkins; 2001. p. 679–710.
78. Viegas GV. Reconstruction of hallux limitus deformity using a first metatarsal sagittal-Z osteotomy. J Foot Ankle Surg 1998;37(3):204–11 [discussion: 261–2].
79. Chang TJ. Stepwise approach to hallux limitus. A surgical perspective. Clin Podiatr Med Surg 1996;13(3):449–59.

Technique and Pearls in Performing the First Metatarsal Phalangeal Joint Arthrodesis

Molly Schnirring-Judge, DPM[a,b,c,d]

KEYWORDS

- First metatarsal phalangeal joint • Arthrodesis
- Fusion techniques • Ankylosis

This article discusses principles of technique with an emphasis on the procedure to prepare a successful first metatarsal phalangeal joint (MTPJ) arthrodesis. The pearls and pitfalls within this article expound on technical nuances including those associated with fixation devices.

CLINICAL CONSIDERATIONS IN 1ST MTPJ ARTHRODESIS

When there is a considerable loss of first MTPJ motion and/or ankylosis is apparent, then a joint preservation procedure may not be feasible. For end-stage degenerative change within the MTPJ, nonreducible joint incongruity, or instability of the first MTPJ, an arthrodesis can provide the most predictable and, arguably, the most definitive correction of the deformity, especially in patients with higher functional demands. In time, numerous modifications in performing arthrodesis of the first MTPJ have been described.[1–17] First MTPJ fusion, whether by traditional or modified techniques, can correct transverse and frontal plane deformity while simultaneously achieving optimal sagittal plane joint position for propulsion when properly executed. This stabilizes the distal aspect of the first ray and, with optimal positioning, improves weight-bearing function of the first MTPJ.

A distinct benefit of this technique is that the ultimate position of the great toe fusion can accommodate a variety of life styles and functional demands. Over time it has been

[a] Cleveland Clinic Foundation- Kaiser Permanente Podiatric Surgical Residency Program, 10 Severence Circle, Cleveland Heights, OH 44070, USA
[b] Ohio University, Firelands Regional Medical Center, Residency Training Program, 111 Hayes Avenue, Sandusky, OH 44870, USA
[c] Graduate Medical Education, Mercy Health Partners, Toledo, OH, USA
[d] Private Practice, North West Ohio Foot and Ankle Institute, LLC, 530 Washington Street, Port Clinton, OH 43452, USA
E-mail address: mjudgemolly@netscape.net

Clin Podiatr Med Surg 28 (2011) 345–359
doi:10.1016/j.cpm.2011.03.001
0891-8422/11/$ – see front matter © 2011 Published by Elsevier Inc.

suggested to position the hallux into slight valgus with mild dorsiflexion in the hope of providing the 10-degrees of dorsiflexion required for propulsion. Experience has shown us to simulate the position of the contra lateral MTPJ. Often a rectus joint position allowing for a fingers breath beneath the hallux tuft is comfortable for locomotion.

It is always prudent to consider the contra lateral 1st ray position and 1st MTPJ alignment in preparing for this procedure. The patient often can confirm with reasonable confidence that they can be satisfied if the joint is positioned similar to that of the opposite foot. This important clinical decision should be discussed with the benefit of a bilateral radiographic exam underlining that the goal is to permanently fix the joint in a position for daily function. There is no greater frustration than to hear a patient ask why their big toe won't move after the fusion has been completed. Failure to achieve optimal position, significant deviation in any plane of motion, can render a solid fusion dysfunctional and painful with every step. Without argument optimal position of fusion and understanding the purpose of the fusion is paramount to success.

If there is any question regarding the perfusion to bone in this region, the benefit of ancillary imaging is warranted. The nuclear medicine triphasic bone scan can provide information on the presence of perfusion deficits as well as the incidence of atrophic or hypertrophic bone especially important in revisional surgery.[18] Magnetic resonance imaging can give insights as to the presence of dysvascular changes in bone, but cannot provide dynamic information regarding active perfusion in the region. As the nuclear medicine bone scan can be scheduled as soon as desired it is considered an efficient, cost effective and useful screening tool that can be supplemented by MRI when necessary.

In considering this procedure, the bone quality and length are scrutinized to determine the potential benefit of incorporating an intercalary bone graft as it may be needed to restore length and provide structural support. This technique involves procurement of a stout autogenous graft when the recipient bed is considered compromised by a deficit in cubic content of bone. Alternately, allogenic bone can be used when bone quality is not an issue. When a nonunion of bone occurs using an allogenic graft the patient may be encouraged to have the procedure revised with the benefit of autogenous graft. For this reason it is becomes infinitely important to educate the patient about the logical options available for grafting prior to the index procedure so that they understand the decision making process. Once the patient understands the risks and benefits of each they can better understand the preferences of their surgeon. The morbidity associated with autogenous tricortical iliac bone grafts has been well established in the literature and should be shared with the patient in advance of surgery.[17]

Whether to use an autograft or allograft implant to provide structural graft and fill voids when preparing joint fusions is an important procedural consideration. This element of surgery has implications that shifts the risk: benefit ratio associated with the procedure. Specifically when considering an autogenous bone graft this ratio shift is in the negative direction and requires a considerable amount of patient education pre operatively. The use of allogenic graft materials while equally important does not shift the risk : benefit ratio to the same extent as it does not carry the potential for donor site morbidity. It is customary to consider the use of a large tricortical-type graft when a structural defect and or significant angular correction was required and in this event an autograft from the iliac crest has been suggested and for many is still preferred.[17,19–22]

Given the research and reports over the past twenty years it has been confirmed that allogenic bone performs well in foot and ankle surgery and can provide excellent functional long-term outcomes. Further the literature suggests that arthrodesing procedures in foot and ankle surgery can be done safely and effectively when using allogenic bone graft materials, sparing the patient a second operative site and avoiding the natural complications attributed to bone graft procurement and host site morbidity.[19,23–25]

While there are instances when arthrodesing procedures can be successful without the benefit of any bone graft[26] there is no replacement for a thorough understanding of the types of bone graft materials available and the function that they provide. (While this section is not geared for the detailed discussion of bone graft materials suggested reading includes the chapter on Bone Grafts in Volume two of the 3rd Edition of the Comprehensive Textbook in Foot and Ankle Surgery.) If bone supplementation is being considered to enhance perfusion to existing bone, then an autogenous graft is perhaps the most physiologic technique.

Whether the fusion is end-to-end or a bone graft is used, the hallmarks for successful bone healing are rigid internal fixation and immobilization of the part.[19,23] The hallmarks for functional success are proper cartilage resection and positioning of the parts accommodating for both fusion and function.[11] **Fig. 1** provides a case study of first MTPJ arthrodesis with long-term follow-up after removal of a silicone implant device secondary to chronic silicone synovitis and recalcitrant pain. The sequence of events begins with the radiographic evaluation including a marker for the primary target of tenderness (see **Fig. 1A**).

TECHNIQUE
Arthrodesis in Hallux Limitus and Failed HAV Surgery

When it is possible to perform a primary end-to-end arthrodesis, meticulous tissue handling and cartilage resection that preserves subchondral bone provides a healthy tissue bed for vascular ingrowth and remineralization of the site. These basic tenants are integral to a successful fusion. In the face of prior HAV surgery, it must be determined whether the original surgical cicatrix location is suitable to provide exposure for this procedure. If the cicatrix lies dorsal or dorsal medial along the first ray segment, then it is probably useful to use that line for incision to minimize the risk of further skin compromise. Should the cicatrix be medial along the joint it can certainly be used if the plan included joint resection followed by a crossing screw technique. If the plan for arthrodesis requires a plate or more complex fixation then further consideration for the incision plan is warranted. Often it is necessary to extend the incision both proximally and distally by an additional 1.0 cm or more to identify normal soft tissue planes and prepare the most meticulous dissection possible for a revision procedure. An incision along the dorsal or dorsal medial aspect of the first metatarsal measuring approximately 6 cm to 8 cm in length allows for adequate exposure of the first MTPJ region, depending on the size of the foot. Sharp and blunt dissection is performed to expose the deep fascia over the joint. The periosteal and capsular incisions are prepared in a linear fashion immediately in line with the skin incision. Once the intra-articular segments are exposed, then thorough denuding of the cartilage surfaces and preparation of the parts for fusion are paramount to establishing a sound foundation for fixation. If a primary arthrodesis is feasible and the metatarsal length is sufficient, then an end-to-end procedure should be completed. Denuding the cartilage from the articular surfaces should be done in a fashion that minimizes bone loss and preserves length, which can be done using rongeurs, curettes, or power instrumentation. Given the natural contours of these small joint surfaces power resection using sagittal saw or cannulated reaming devices are often the most effective and efficient. Denuding surfaces that are deeply concave or concavoconvex are challenging to

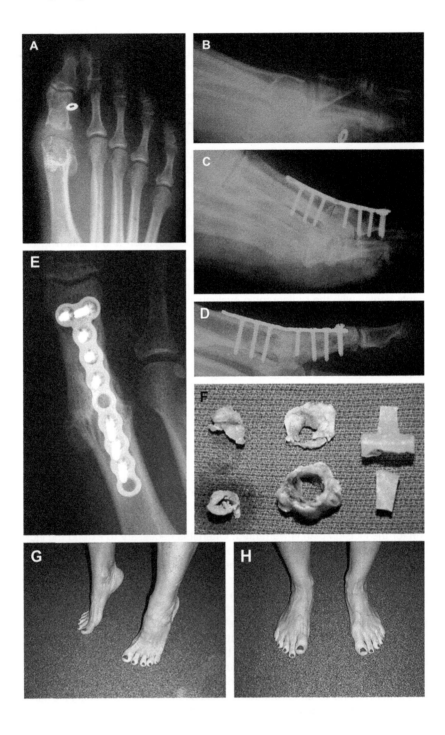

prepare with manual instrumentation alone and leave room for error when resecting the most deep recesses of the site. A crescentic blade can be used to resect the cartilage with a minimum of bone loss and follows the natural contours of the articulation preserving structure and congruence. An alternate technique uses a cone reamer and contours the surfaces to preserve the ball-and-socket configuration. The technique used should be whichever is most comfortable and expeditious for the surgeon. The desired morphology of the fusion site is reliant on the resection technique; if the ball-and-socket configuration is to be maintained, then curettage, conical reamer, or crescentic saw blade resection will facilitate that goal (**Fig. 2**). These techniques tend to result in the least bone loss and therefore aid in preserving the final length of the first ray. If a flush-cut, flat, end-to-end arthrodesis is desired, then resection using a fine-tooth, sagittal saw is preferred to minimize bone loss. This method creates a ginglymus-shaped joint that allows for 2 points of fixation using pins, screws, staples, or circlage techniques. Although rongeurs can be used for this purposed, they are difficult to use on the concave surface of the hallux base, especially in dense or sclerotic bone. Copious irrigation is completed before realignment of the parts to remove any bone debris that may interfere with bone apposition. Additional

---

Fig. 1. (*A*) Dorsoplantar radiograph Preoperative view of the profound cystic degeneration resulting from a total first MTPJ silicone implant. The metallic marker indicates the region of osseous insufficiency as the silicone began to erode through the phalanx in this region, resulting in the target area of pain. The sclerotic margins about the implant and increased soft tissue density about the joint are easily appreciated. (*B*) Lateral radiograph. This preoperative view of the distal portion of the silicone implant is subluxed dorsally and the implant has eroded against the inferior margin of the phalanx. The metallic marker indicates the target of irritation on weight bearing. The flexion deformity of the hallux is easily appreciated because the dorsal subluxation of the implant has given the flexor hallucis longus a mechanical advantage. (*C*) Lateral radiograph showing the interpositional bone graft required to restore length because of a complication of HAV surgery. The low-profile titanium plate stabilizes the graft-arthrodesis interfaces. In this procedure, each interface is at risk for bone healing complication such as nonunion compared with an end-to-end arthrodesis in which there is only 1 site at risk. The proximal aspect of the graft-metatarsal interface is easily appreciated as a vertical lucency in this early postoperative view. (*D*) Lateral radiograph. At 4 years after surgery, complete incorporation of the graft is easily appreciated. There is approximately 20 degrees of dorsiflexion in the hallux position to allow for the athletic activity of this physical therapist. There is an increased prominence of the most distal screws. Removal of the entire construct would take place once complete bone union has been confirmed and sufficient clinical progress merits removal of these devices. At 4 years after the index procedure, this younger physical therapist elected to have the devices removed and began aggressive rehabilitation within the following 2 weeks. (*E*) Dorsoplantar radiograph. At 4 years after surgery the graft is indistinguishable from natural bone beneath this low-profile titanium plate. The minimal profile of this modular hand plate makes it well tolerated even after 4 years of heavy athletic activity. (*F*) Gross pathology specimens. The remnants of the total joint silicone implant and thickened rings of fibrinous ingrowths are excised before curettement of the medullary contents of bone. (*G*) Clinical examination to include toe rise maneuvers are performed with ease 10 years after first MTPJ arthrodesis using a very low-profile plate (Synthes North America). Before surgery, the patient was unable to bear weight on the first MTPJ and suffered from lateral overloading and metatarsal stress fracture syndrome. (*H*) The right foot as a well-healed cicatrix that is flush with the surrounding tissues. There is no evidence of irritation about the soft tissue sleeve and the patient is able to perform her daily activities and continues to be highly athletic.

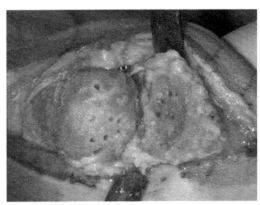

Fig. 2. The articular surfaces of the first MTPJ have been denuded while preserving the subchondral surface. Once fenestrated using a 1.5-mm wire pass drill bit, the parts can be juxtaposed for arthrodesis. Several techniques can be used to denude cartilage from these articular surfaces with minimum bone loss, such as curettage, the use of crescentic saw blades, and curettement or the use of conical reamers. (*Courtesy of* Jordan P. Grossman, DPM, Akron, OH.)

fenestration of the subchondral region of bone using a 0.54 K-wire or 1.5 mm wire pass drill bit and may be desired if this layer is very thick or sclerotic. This fenestration encourages immediate perfusion and in time facilitates vascular ingrowths.

Once the bone has been prepared for arthrodesis, the position of fusion must be determined; this is the most important functional decision to be made during the procedure. During surgery, it is possible to simulate weight bearing by flexing the patient's knee and placing the foot at 90 degrees to the leg with the foot flat on a solid surface (eg, an instrument tray lid). With the ankle at 90 degrees and the foot in neutral weight-bearing position, the hallux can be elevated just until it is possible to pass an index finger freely between the hallux and the tray. This subtle dorsiflexion of the hallux allows enough motion to load and propulse off the hallux interphalangeal joint (HIPJ). With the hallux rectus or slightly abducted to parallel the adjacent digit, the position should be comfortable in sensible shoe gear. This intra operative exercise also serves to prevent an equinated position of the hallux. Although a wide range of positions have been suggested as optimal for a first MTPJ arthrodesis, generally the desired position of fusion is considered to be 15 degrees to 25 degrees of dorsiflexion with a similar degree of abduction, often 15 degrees to 20 degrees.[27] This position of fusion takes into account that the first MTPJ must dorsiflex approximately 20 degrees to accommodate a 2.5-cm heel height.[28–30] Although these parameters are a general guideline, position of the fusion site becomes a function of the surgeon's experience and preference. Some would recommend creating a congruous first MTPJ with only slight elevation and abduction as is this authors preference. Once adequate joint position and alignment have been achieved, provisional fixation should be applied. Temporary fixation of the parts using one or two 0.062 K-wires should be placed to firmly capture the desired position and intraoperative radiographs should confirm final position, alignment, and adequate coaptation of the parts. Multiple orthogonal planes should be reviewed to ensure that a maximum of bone-to-bone contact has been achieved. Once satisfied with position and alignment, the decision to use crossing K-wire fixation or alternate techniques to provide rigid internal fixation can be made. Fixation should be critically assessed to ensure that there are no devices interfering with HIPJ joint function and that no device is protruding plantarly to impede weight bearing.

Internal fixation for an end-to-end arthrodesis is a matter of surgeon preference in good-quality bone. Crossing K-wires work well for osteoporosis, although other K-wire configurations have proved equally effective. Parallel 0.062 K-wires or small Steinman pins can be used as external devices running out of the hallux base and ret-rograded into the first metatarsal, and can be removed after solid bone union has been achieved (**Fig. 3**A). Given the inherent size and shape of this articulation there is a rela-tively small volume of bone to coapt and compress and so a simple approach to 1st MTPJ arthrodesis and arguably the most common is the use of a single oblique screw or crossing compression screw technique as seen in **Fig. 3**B and C. The use of an interfragmentary screw and a low-profile titanium plate is useful in younger patients and otherwise in patients with dense bone **Fig. 3**D. Demonstrates the interfragmentary screw and low profile titanium plate technique side by side with the radiograph of the same **Fig. 3**E. The plate may be placed either dorsally or medially across the joint, and placement can vary depending on available soft tissue coverage. When the dorsal skin has suffered from atrophy and considerable adhesion exists, the vascularity of the region may not support a dorsal plate and the medial application is a viable alternative. The use of plates and screws, threaded Steinman pins, K-wire and circlage, single oblique screw, and double crossing screw techniques, as well as the peg-and-hole technique, have all been described with successful outcomes.[6,7,9,10,12,13,15,29,31–53] With the advent of locking plates, these devices have entered everyday practice when dealing with severely osteopenic or osteoporotic bone. Demineralized bone may be evident, caused by chronic systemic disease (such as diabetes, rheumatoid arthritis, and malabsorption syndromes), trauma, disuse osteopenia secondary to long-term impairment, or from osteoporosis. In these cases, it is prudent to pursue not only the benefit of a low-profile device but a locking device to enhance the long-term stability of the construct. The transition from non–weight bearing to weight bearing has traditionally been a tenuous time in the rehabilitation process and, with current technology, locking plate systems have provided enhanced stability and instilled a higher degree of confidence in that advancement (**Fig. 4**). Regardless of the devices used to fixate the site of bone union, there is no substitute for using the basic principles in the AO (Arbeitsgemeinschaft für Osteosynthese fragen) technique to align, coapt, compress, and stabilize the parts.

Once satisfied with the position and alignment of the fusion and internal fixation device(s), copious irrigation is completed and a layered closure is performed. Care is taken to cover the periosteum over the fixation devices to prevent irritation from prom-inent devices or interference with the function of the extensor tendons. A sterile bandaging of the foot and ankle is completed with the benefit of a Jones compression dressing incorporating a cryotherapy unit as desired. A posterior splint or a fiberglass eggshell can be applied to encourage compliance with the non–weight-bearing requirement. The postoperative course is a matter of debate. Traditionally, a non–weight-bearing course for 4 to 6 weeks has been exercised, whereas others suggest modified, protected weight bearing in a firm sole or OrthoWedge shoe. Regardless of the technique used, the site of fusion should be protected and monitored clinically and radiographically for 6 to 8 weeks to ensure adequate bone consolidation and main-tenance of position. The physical rehabilitation plan includes a short-leg compression stocking beginning once the surgical wound has completely healed. This stocking prevents prolonged edema and the development of subsequent neuritic symptoms. Gradual advancement into firm-soled athletic shoe gear is pursued to tolerance as early as 6 weeks after surgery if radiographic consolidation is evident on multiple views.

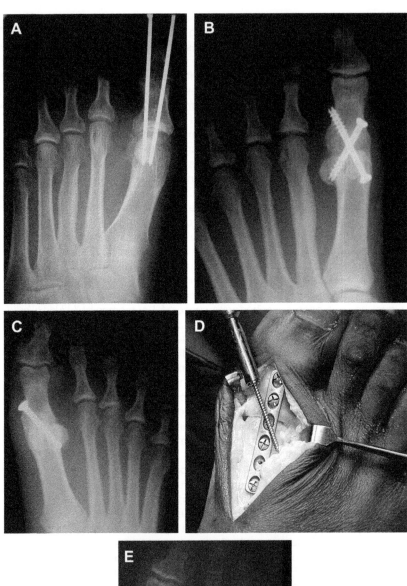

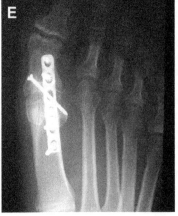

PEARLS/PITFALLS
Modification of the First MTPJ Arthrodesis

The technique of creating a peg-and-hole arthrodesis construct has proved efficacious even as a primary surgery to correct the HAV deformity. When an overaggressive exostectomy has been performed and the residual metatarsal head has been reduced to a fraction of its original morphology, this technique may prove curative.[53] The authors declare an 85% success rate, with the caveat that it is suggested for elderly patients. It is claimed that the peg-and-hole technique does not require internal fixation and that protected weight bearing is allowed to tolerance, as opposed to traditional protocols associated with first MTPJ arthrodesis. Of the 31 patients undergoing this technique for severe HAV deformity, none experienced hallux varus even when significant metatarsus primus varus was evident after surgery. In the original article, the technique was described using a beef bone peg and manual impaction of the parts without fixation and was performed in 33 cases, resulting in a 90% fusion rate.[53] Of the 10% that experienced nonunion, the peg was broken at the fusion site when resuming unprotected weight bearing at 6 weeks (8 weeks after surgery). The original investigator suggested prolonged plaster cast immobilization for 8 to 10 weeks, contrary to more contemporary recommendations by Humbert and colleagues[37] 20 years later.

A similar technique, using specially designed reamers, fashions a cone at the metatarsal head for a peg-and-socket articulation. After reviewing 85 such first MTPJ fusions in a 20-year period, the investigators reported a 97.6% fusion rate while maintaining the corrected position in long-term follow-up.[35]

Intercalary bone graft

Using preoperative radiographs is the best way to predict the extent of bone deficits caused by devitalized bone and to prepare for the size of bone graft required for harvest. The size of the graft must be sufficient to fill the defect and restore optimal length to the first ray segment. Once the size of the graft is determined, selection of the size and shape of the plate can be completed. This preoperative assessment allows precise measures of the length of the plate and allows estimation of the length of the screws required along each segment of the ray. To interpose an intercalary bone graft, it is beneficial to first measure the plate against the entire length of the metatarsal bone graft/phalangeal base segment to determine where the center of the plate should

◄─────────────────────────────────────

Fig 3. (A) Radiograph of the parallel Steinman pin technique. Notice how the joint is coapted and compressed in congruous alignment and that the ball and socket configuration of the joint has been maintained despite cartilage resection. (B) Shown here the crossing compression screw technique using partially threaded cannulated screws. Notice that the bone has been sufficiently compressed and consolidated that the separation between the parts is no longer visible. The stress fracture noted within the 2nd metatarsal is a consequence of faulty mechanics that occurred prior to the time of arthrodesis. With a stable 1st MTPJ fusion this region of bone will remodel over time. (C) Use of the single oblique compression screw technique seen here with a standard fully threaded cortical screw achieving complete consolidation of the fusion site. These simple techniques (A–C) are by far and away the most favored when undertaking an end to end 1st MTPJ fusion in healthy bone. (D) Intra operative view of a low profile plate used with the benefit of an interfragmentary screw. The length of the screw is compared to the fusion site prior to placement. In this instance the screw will be used as a positional device while the plate is applied using an eccentric drilling technique to afford compression across the site of fusion. This combination technique results in a stable arthrodesis and provides excellent bone consolidation and long term function as seen in the follow up radiograph (E).

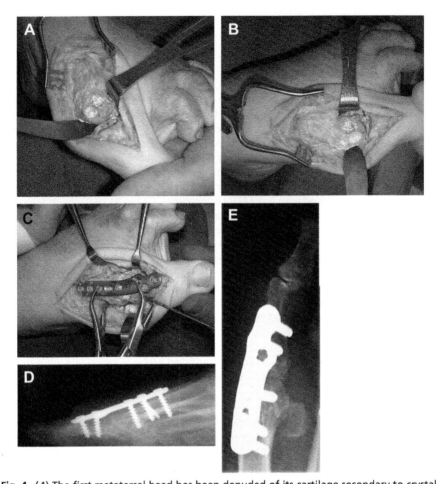

Fig. 4. (*A*) The first metatarsal head has been denuded of its cartilage secondary to crystalline induced arthropathy; chronic hyper uricemia . The enlarged erosive changes are a hallmark for this disease. The systemic disease denuded the metatarsal head of its normal chondral surface. The generalized osteopenia secondary to long standing diabetes and chronic gout makes this a good candidate for the use of a customized locking plate designed especially for the first MTPJ. This construct will withstand the high demands of this neuropathic and obese female as she resumes full weight bearing activities of daily living. (*B*) Cavernous defects remain in the distal segment of the metatarsal head and can be filled using autogenous or allogenic graft materials as desired to fill voids and improve the bone bed quality. The degenerative disease had removed most of the chondral surface allowing for manual debridement of the 1st MTPJ preserving the ball-and-socket morphology without the need for special reamers. Note the thickened periosteum that remains intact just proximal to the metatarsal neck region, which is a secondary effect residual from the combination of hyperglycemia and hyperuricemia. (*C*) Given the presence of generalized osteopenia in the face of chronic diabetes mellitus and gout, the use of a locking plate is warranted. Note the star-shaped holes designed to accommodate locking screws, and the centrally located rectangula hole that allows the use of standard screws, as desired seen in *C* (VLP® FOOT MTP Fusion Plate from Smith & Nephew, Inc). The holes on either side of the fusion site can be drilled eccentrically to provide compression in the event that an interfragmentary screw is not used. Follow up 1st MTPJ arthrodesis using the locking plate technique. Notice that the plate provides axial compression while the eccentric drilling technique allowed for compression across the site of fusion. Seen here is the 3-month follow up plain film views medial oblique (*D*) and lateral views (*E*). Notice that the compressed joint can be appreciated in both views. No evidence of resorptive change or migration of fixation devices. The small oblique screw seen in the background of the lateral view represents a previous 2nd metatarsal osteotomy performed elsewhere.

lie. It is desirable to have at least 2 or 3 points of fixation proximal and distal to the graft to create the most stable construct whenever possible. When using the small, low-profile devices designed for the small bones of the foot, this may require the use of a 10-hole plate or larger. On the back table, the graft can be prepared by running a single screw through the plate and graft to create a preliminary strut for mounting the plate to the site of fusion. With the plate and graft secured, this solid unit can be interposed between the metatarsal and the phalangeal base. Compression of the plate along the first ray is achieved with the benefit of plate clamps while the remaining screws are placed using standard A-O technique. To provide compression across the fusion site, eccentric drilling of the screws placed just proximal and distal to the graft should be performed.

Bone graft for the first MTPJ arthrodesis: allogenic versus autogenous

Whether to use an autograft or allograft implant has been a matter of debate in recent years, and there has been a lot of research to investigate the question. Traditionally, when a large tricortical-type graft was desired, an autograft from the iliac crest was preferred.[20–22,54]

Allogenic bone performs well in foot and ankle surgery and can provide excellent functional long-term outcomes. The current literature suggests that arthrodesing procedures in foot and ankle surgery can be done safely and effectively with the benefit of allogenic bone graft materials, sparing the patient a second operative site and avoiding the natural complications attributed to bone graft procurement.[19,23–25]

Arthrodesing procedures can be successful even without the benefit of any bone graft.[26,28,55] If bone supplementation is being considered strictly to enhance perfusion at the arthrodesis site, then an autogenous graft is the most physiologic technique.

When considering bone grafting in the small bones of the fore foot, the discussion differs dramatically from that in rear foot arthrodesing procedures. In large bone reconstruction, the use of autogenous bone remains the graft material of choice in arthrodesing procedures.[19] However, despite its inherent lack of bone morphogenic protein, allogenic bone graft has been shown to perform well in numerous procedures in foot and ankle surgery.[23] When given a healthy perigraft environment, these bone bank specimens provide ample structural support and a porous surface area to allow for creeping substitution in secondary bone healing.[56] In contrast to this, it has been shown that autogenous bone graft is preferred in salvage reconstruction of the very small bones of the fore foot where vascular compromise in the adjacent tissue beds is an issue.[57] Most investigators agree that, if there is any question of the vascular competence of the recipient bed or the peripheral graft sites, then the benefits of using autogenous grafting to enhance bone healing outweigh the risks associated with donor site morbidity.[23,56,58–61]

Techniques in autogenous bone grafting of the first MTPJ have been suggested specifically when length has been lost after metatarsal osteotomy procedures.[62] Single-stage lengthening techniques using autogenous bone graft have been compared with the callus distraction technique. Ultimately, it is reported that the single-stage approach yields bone healing at a faster rate (6 vs 10.8 weeks respectively in one study). Neither technique resulted in neurovascular compromise, with similar outcomes in length achieved from both.[63] The use of intercalary bone grafting in revisional bunion surgery to restore length has been documented with good success even in cases in which bone quality was suspect.[20,21] In the case of hallux rigidus length and even bone quality may not be an issue and so bone graft remains a viable adjunct for arthrodesis in these cases but typically is not required.

Whether the fusion is end-to-end or a bone graft is used, the hallmark to successful bone healing is rigid internal fixation and immobilization of the parts. The hallmark of functional success is proper joint preparation and positioning of the parts for fusion and function. Based upon published reports in large-series reviews of first MTPJ arthrodesis procedures, the union rate ranges from 68% to 100%.[6,7,9,10,12,13,15,29,31–35,37,38,40–43,45–50,52] As many of these procedures were performed for failed hallux abducto valgus (HAV) surgery, HAV and hallux rigidus (HR) these statistics underline the predictability and reproducibility of the technique. When a bone graft is used, it is intuitive that the complication rate in bone healing may be increased; however, this was not borne out in the review mentioned earlier, as only 1 study reported the use of bone grafting (the in lay technique specifically) and reported a union rate of 97%. A prospective review of strictly first MTPJ fusion using interpositional bone graft would be the most valuable of evidence based studies to complete this discussion and to date this information is lacking.

Further considerations in fixation for the first MTPJ arthrodesis

Even when an overly aggressive exostectomy or modified cheilectomy has been performed, it does not usually affect the length pattern of the first ray and commonly leaves the foundation for a straightforward arthrodesis. Stabilization of the construct can then be prepared definitively using a variety of techniques depending on the quality of bone present. In the event of osteoporosis, modifications in the fixation plan may include the crossing K-wire technique (with or without the prebending), dual or triple parallel external K-wire technique (see **Fig. 3**), staples (2-staple technique using 90 degree staple orientations), or the use of a locking plate. With unusually porous bone, the use of at least 2 points of fixation is advised to prevent motion about the fusion site, and the benefits of a locking plate in these instances cannot be overemphasized.

When normal bone quality exists, aside from the eminence deficit, then more traditional devices can be used to provide an end-to-end arthrodesis, and these include single- screw or double-screw techniques, staples, or the combination of circlage and 0.062 K-wire.

REFERENCES

1. Flavin R, Stephens MM. Arthrodesis of the first metatarsophalangeal joint using a dorsal titanium contoured plate. Foot Ankle Int 2004;25(11):783–7.
2. Calderone DR, Wertheimer SJ. First metatarsophalangeal joint arthrodesis using a mini-Hoffman external fixator. J Foot Ankle Surg 1993;32:517–25.
3. Shim GS, Pikscher I, Frankel N. First metatarsophalangeal joint arthrodesis with a truncated cone reamer system. J Foot Surg 1992;31:342–9.
4. Bouche RT, Adad JR. Arthrodesis of the first metatarsophalangeal joint in active people. Clin Podiatr Med Surg 1996;13:461–84.
5. Yu GV, Shook JE. Arthrodesis of the first metatarsophalangeal joint: current recommendations. J Am Podiatr Med Assoc 1994;84:266–80.
6. Chana GS, Andrew TA, Cotteril CP. A simple method of arthrodesis of the first metatarsophalangeal joint. J Bone Joint Surg Br 1984;66:703–5.
7. Coughlin MJ. Arthrodesis of the first metatarsophalangeal joint with mini fragment plate fixation. Orthopedics 1990;13:1037–44.
8. Holmes GB Jr. Arthrodesis of the first metatarsophalangeal joint using interfragmentary screw and plate. Foot Ankle 1992;13:333–5.
9. Marin GA. Arthrodesis of the first metatarsophalangeal joint of the big toe for hallux valgus and hallux rigidus; a new method. Int Surg 1968;50:175–80.

10. Phillips J, Hooper G. A simple technique for arthrodesis of the first metatarsopha-langeal joint. J Bone Joint Surg Br 1986;68:774–5.
11. Smith RW, Joanis TL, Maxwell PD. Great toe metatarsophalangeal joint arthrod-esis: a user friendly technique. Foot Ankle 1992;13:367–77.
12. Turan I, Lindgren U. Compression screw arthrodesis of the first metatarsophalan-geal joint of the foot. Clin Orthop 1987;221:292–5.
13. Wilson JN. Cone arthrodesis of the first metatarsophalangeal joint. J Bone Joint Surg Br 1967;49:98–101.
14. Wilson CL. A method of fusion of the metatarsophalangeal joint of the great toe. J Bone Joint Surg Am 1958;40:384–5.
15. Wu KK. Arthrodesis of the first metatarsophalangeal joint of the great toe with Herbert screws: a clinical analysis of 27 cases. J Foot Ankle Surg 1993;32:47–52.
16. Kupcha PC, Fitzpatrick MJ. Application of the tension band technique for arthrod-esis of the fore foot and mid foot. Foot Ankle Int 1996;17:784.
17. DeOrio JK, Farber DC. Morbidity associated with anterior iliac crest bone grafting in foot and ankle surgery. Foot Ankle Int 2005;26(2):147–51.
18. Jacobs AM, Klein S, Oloff L, et al. Radionuclide evaluation of complications after metatarsal osteotomy and implant arthroplasty of the foot. J Foot Surg 1984;23:86–96.
19. McGarvey WC, Braly WG. Bone graft in hind foot arthrodesis: allograft versus autograft. Orthopedics 1996;19(5):389–94.
20. Brodsky JW, Ptaszek AJ, Morris SG. Salvage first MTP arthrodesis utilizing ICBG: clinical evaluation and outcome. Foot Ankle Int 2000;21(4):290–6.
21. Myerson MS, Schon LC, McGuigan FX, et al. Result of arthrodesis of the hallux metatarsophalangeal joint using bone graft for restoration of length. Foot Ankle Int 2000;21(4):297–306.
22. Brown CH. A technique for distal tibial bone graft for arthrodesis of the foot and ankle. Foot Ankle Int 2000;21(9):780–1.
23. Mahan KT, Hillstrom HJ. Bone grafting in foot and ankle surgery. A review of 300 cases. J Am Podiatr Med Assoc 1998;88(3):109–18.
24. Pietrzak WS, Perns SV, Keyes J, et al. Demineralized bone matrix graft: a scientific and clinical case study assessment. J Foot Ankle Surg 2005;44(5):345–53.
25. Chou LB, Halligan BW. Treatment of severe, painful pes planovalgus deformity with hindfoot arthrodesis and wedge-shaped tricortical allograft. Foot Ankle Int 2007;28(5):569–74.
26. Rosenfeld PF, Budgen SA, Saxby TS. Triple arthrodesis: is bone grafting neces-sary? The results in 100 consecutive cases. J Bone Joint Surg Br 2005;87(2):175–8.
27. Yu GV, Schnirring-Judge M, Shook JE. Complications of hallux abducto valgus surgery. In: Banks AS, Downey MS, Martin DE, Miller SJ, editors. McGlamry's compre-hensive textbook of foot and ankle surgery. 3rd edition. Philadelphia: Lippincott Williams & Wilkins; 2001. p. 655–77.
28. Weinraub GM, Cheung C. Efficacy of allogenic bone implants in a series of consecutive elective foot procedures. J Foot Ankle Surg 2003;42(2):86–9.
29. Sussman RE, Russo CL, Marquit H, et al. Arthrodesis of the first metatarsophalan-geal joint. J Am Podiatr Med Assoc 1986;76:631–5.
30. Sussman RE, D'Amico JC. The influence of the height of the heel on the fist meta-tarsophalangeal joint. J Am Podiatry Assoc 1984;74:504.
31. Harrison MH, Harvey FJ. Arthrodesis of the first metatarsophalangeal joint for hallux valgus and rigidus. J Bone Joint Surg Am 1963;45:471–80.

32. Moynihan F. Arthrodesis of the first metatarsophalangeal joint of the great toe. J Bone Joint Surg Br 1967;49:544–51.
33. Fitzgerald JA. A review of results of arthrodesis of the first metatarsophalangeal joint. J Bone Joint Surg Br 1969;51:488–93.
34. Raymakers R, Waugh W. The treatment of metatarsalgia with hallux valgus. J Bone Joint Surg Br 1971;53:684.
35. Wilkinson J. Cone arthrodesis of the first metatarsophalangeal joint. Acta Orthop Scand 1978;49:267. p. 627–30.
36. McKeever D. Arthrodesis of the fist metatarsophalangeal joint for hallux valgus, hallux rigidus and metatarsus primus varus. J Bone Joint Surg Am 1952;34:129–34.
37. Humbert JL, Bourbonniere C, Laurin CA. Metatarsophalangeal joint fusion for hallux valgus: indications and effect on the first metatarsal ray. Can Med Assoc J 1979;120:937–56.
38. Von Salis-Soglio G, Thoners W. Arthrodesis of the first metatarsophalangeal joint of the great toe. Arch Orthop Trauma Surg 1979;95:7.
39. Mann RA, Oates JC. Arthrodesis of the first metatarsophalangeal joint. Foot Ankle 1980;1:159–66.
40. Riggs SA, Johnson EW. McKeever arthrodesis for the painful hallux. Foot Ankle 1983;3:248–53.
41. Johannson JE, Barrington TW. Cone arthrodesis of the first metatarsophalangeal joint. Foot Ankle 1984;4:244–8.
42. Beauchamp CG, Kirby T, Rudge SR, et al. Fusion of the first metatarsophalangeal joint in fore foot arthroplasty. Clin Orthop 1984;190:249–53.
43. Mann RA, Thompson FM. Arthrodesis of the first metatarsophalangeal joint for hallux valgus in rheumatoid arthritis. J Bone Joint Surg Am 1984;55:687–92.
44. Coughlin MJ, Mann RA. Arthrodesis of the first metatarsophalangeal joint as a salvage for the failed Keller procedure. J Bone Joint Surg Am 1987;69:68–74.
45. Mann RA, Katcherian DA. Relationship of metatarsophalangeal joint fusion on the intermetatarsal angle. Foot Ankle 1989;10:8–11.
46. Gregory JL, Childers R, Higgins KR, et al. Arthrodesis of the first metatarsophalangeal joint: a review of the literature and long term retrospective analysis. J Foot Surg 1990;29:369–74.
47. O'Doherty DP, Lowrey LG, Magnussen PA, et al. The management of the painful first metatarsophalangeal joint in the older patient. J Bone Joint Surg Br 1990;72:839.
48. Lampe HIH, Fonteije P, van Linje B. Weight bearing after arthrodesis of the first metatarsophalangeal joint: a randomized study of 61 cases. Acta Orthop Scand 1991;62:544–5.
49. Hughes J, Grace D, Clark P, et al. Metatarsal head excision for rheumatoid arthritis: 4-year follow up of 68 feet with and without hallux fusion. Acta Orthop Scand 1991;62:63.
50. Niskanen RO, Lehtimaki MY, Hamalainen MM, et al. Arthrodesis of the first metatarsophalangeal joint in rheumatoid arthritis. Acta Orthop Scand 1993;64:100–2.
51. Wu KK. First metatarsophalangeal joint fusion in the salvage of failed hallux abducto valgus operations. J Foot Ankle Surg 1994;33:383–95.
52. Hecht PJ, Gibbons MJ, Wapner KL, et al. Arthrodesis of the first metatarsophalangeal joint to salvage failed silicone implant arthroplasty. Foot Ankle Int 1997;18:383–90.
53. Tupman GS. Bone peg arthrodesis of the first metatarso-phalangeal joint. Postgrad Med J 1959;35:583–6.

54. Raikin SM, Brislin K. Local bone graft harvested from the distal tibia or calcaneus for surgery of the foot and ankle. Foot Ankle Int 2005;26(6):449–53.
55. Myerson MS, Neufeld SK, Uribe J. Fresh-frozen structural allografts in the foot and ankle. J Bone Joint Surg Am 2005;87(1):113–20.
56. Catanzariti A, Karlock L. Application of allograft bone in foot and ankle surgery. J Foot Ankle Surg 1996;35:440–51.
57. Mahan KT. Bone graft reconstruction of a flail digit. J Am Podiatr Med Assoc 1992;82(5):264–8.
58. Mann RA. Calcaneal donor bone grafts. J Am Podiatr Med Assoc 1994;84:1–9.
59. Philip AJ. Bone grafts: autogenous vs. allogenic/cortical vs. cancellous. In: Dinapoli DR, editor. Reconstructive surgery of the foot and leg: update 1990. Tucker (GA): The Podiatry Institute; 1990. p. 120–3.
60. Mahan KT. Bone grafts materials and perioperative management. In: Camasta CA, editor. Reconstructive surgery of the foot and leg: update '95. Tucker (GA): The Podiatry Institute; 1995. p. 69–75.
61. Mahan KT, Downey MS, Weinfield GD. Autogenous bone graft interpositional arthrodesis for the correction of flail toe. A retrospective analysis of 22 cases. J Am Podiatr Med Assoc 2003;93(3):167–73.
62. Kaplan EG, Kaplan GS. Metatarsal lengthening by use of autogenous bone graft and internal wire compression fixation: a preliminary report. J Foot Surg 1978; 17(2):60–6.
63. Choi IH, Chung MS, Baek GH, et al. Metatarsal lengthening in congenital brachy-metatarsia: one-stage lengthening versus lengthening by callotasis. J Pediatr Orthop 1999;19(5):660–4.

Modern Techniques in Hallux Rigidus Surgery

William T. DeCarbo, DPM, AACFAS[a,b,*], Jeffrey Lupica, DPM[c],
Christopher F. Hyer, DPM[a]

KEYWORDS

- Hallux rigidus • Osteoarthritis • MTP • Cheilectomy
- Arthroplasty

The first metatarsophalangeal (MTP) joint plays a significant role in the normal function of the foot and its function in the gait cycle. Pain and decreased motion of the first metatarsal joint makes normal ambulation and propulsion difficult. Hallux rigidus or osteoarthritis (OA) of the first MTP joint is a condition that causes pain and stiffness in the joint. This condition was first described as a plantar-flexed position of the proximal phalanx relative to the metatarsal head by Davies-Colley[1] in 1887 and termed hallux flexus. Cotterill[2] later coined the term hallux rigidus while describing the same condition. Hallux rigidus often presents with osteophyte formation around the joint, with eventual loss of articular cartilage and osteolysis. OA of the first MTP joint is a debilitating affliction of the great toe and the most common form of degeneration in the foot affecting 35% to 60% of the population older than 65 years.[3,4] The terms hallux limitus and hallux rigidus have been used interchangeably to describe this condition, with hallux rigidus representing the end-stage form of this arthritis resulting in ankylosis.[5] Other than hallux valgus, hallux rigidus is the most common disorder the first MTP joint, often leading to more disability.[6,7]

Daily activities such as walking, running, stair climbing, and squatting become difficult as the arthritic disease progresses. Coughlin and Shurnas[8] indicated that the average age of onset of symptoms was 43 years and the average age of surgical intervention was 50 years. Initial conservative treatment includes the use of nonsteroidal antiinflammatory drugs (NSAIDs), modifications in shoe gear, and custom molded orthotics. However, for many patients, these treatments do not provide permanent relief of symptoms. Surgical intervention is usually warranted in the later stages of

Disclosure: William T. DeCarbo, DPM, is a Consultant for Extremity Medical.
[a] Orthopedic Foot and Ankle Center, 300 Polaris Parkway Suite 2000, Westerville, OH 43082, USA
[b] The Orthopedic Group, 800 Plaza Drive, Suite 140, Belle Vernon, PA 15012, USA
[c] Department of Podiatric Medicine and Surgery, Kaiser Permanente/Cleveland Clinic Foundation, Kaiser Permanente/Cleveland Clinic, 9500 Euclid Avenue, Cleveland, OH 44195, USA
* Corresponding author. Orthopedic Foot and Ankle Center, OhioHealth, 300 Polaris Parkway Suite 2000, Westerville, OH 43082.
E-mail address: ofacresearch@orthofootankle.com

Clin Podiatr Med Surg 28 (2011) 361–383
doi:10.1016/j.cpm.2011.02.001   **podiatric.theclinics.com**

the deformity. Surgical options include arthroplasty, implant arthroplasty, and arthrodesis, among others.

ETIOLOGY/PATHOPHYSIOLOGY

The cause of hallux rigidus is not completely understood and considered by many to be multifactorial. Several risk factors including age, sex, trauma, systemic arthropathies, hypermobile first ray, metatarsus primus elevatus, short or long first metatarsal, family history, and ill-fitting shoes have been proposed.[5,9–16] Nilsonne[5] proposed that a long first metatarsal increases the stress at the first MTP joint during propulsion, whereas Lambrinudi[17] theorized that an elevated first metatarsal leads to flexion contracture of the first MTP joint. Several studies found no correlation between hallux rigidus and first metatarsal elevation.[3,18]

Hindfoot valgus has also been proposed as a related and possible cause for the pathologic condition. A retrospective cohort study of 1592 patients over a 13-year period showed an association between hindfoot valgus and the development of OA of the first MTP joint.[19] The investigators showed a 23% more likelihood to develop first MTP joint OA in patients with hindfoot valgus.

A recent study by Zammit and colleagues[20] reviewed the literature across several databases to identify and analyze demographic and structural factors associated with hallux limitus and rigidus. They concluded that a dorsiflexed first metatarsal relative to the second metatarsal, plantar-flexed forefoot on the hindfoot, wider first metatarsal and proximal phalanx, and longer hallux and longer medial and lateral sesamoids predispose the first MTP joint to compression during the propulsion phase of gait that may lead to hallux limitus or rigidus.

Coughlin and Shurnas[21] reported hallux rigidus being associated with hallux interphalangeus and the female gender. An association with familial history for bilateral hallux rigidus and history of trauma for unilateral hallux rigidus was found. The investigators also reported that a flat or chevron-shaped MTP joint was more common in these patients. Trauma, from either an isolated injury or repetitive microtrauma, remains the most common cause reported in the literature for hallux rigidus.[22]

CLINICAL/RADIOGRAPHIC PRESENTATION

Patients with hallux rigidus commonly present with pain and/or stiffness at the first MTP joint that worsens with activity, barefoot walking, or soft-sole shoes. The pain is typically an aching sensation deep within the joint. This pain is often localized to the dorsal aspect of the joint early in the disease, becoming more diffuse with progression.[23] In advanced stages with bony exostosis, the dorsal soft tissues may be irritated by shoe wear (**Fig. 1**). This dorsal irritation may cause paresthesia or numbness of the medial dorsal cutaneous nerve as it courses over the medial hallux. Lateral foot pain may be experienced because of compensation of the gait cycle while the patient tries to offload the first MTP joint.

Objectively, patients present with a tender, swollen joint with motion of the first MTP joint restricted, especially with the foot loaded. Restriction of motion with the foot loaded is termed functional hallux limitus/rigidus. Decreased motion without the foot loaded is termed structural hallux limitus/rigidus. This distinction gives some indication of the cause of the disease. Pain or callus formation at the plantar interphalangeal joint of the hallux is also common with restricted first MTP motion.[24] Pain with joint manipulation may be elicited and end range of motion (dorsiflexion or plantarflexion) or midrange with extensive cartilage loss of the first MTP joint.

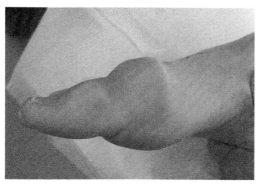

Fig. 1. Advanced stage of hallux rigidus.

Anteroposterior (AP), lateral, and oblique radiographs in the weight-bearing position should be obtained. The AP radiograph often shows asymmetric joint space narrowing with sclerosis, subchondral cysts, and widening and flattening of the first metatarsal head (**Figs. 2** and **3**). The lateral radiograph often reveals a dorsal metatarsal osteophyte with loose bone fragments (joint mouse) (**Fig. 4**). There have been multiple classification systems to describe hallux rigidus (**Figs. 5–7**).[25] Although there exists no clear construction of classification systems for hallux rigidus, 2 systems, most often based on radiographic and clinical parameters, are used. Hattrup and Johnson[26]

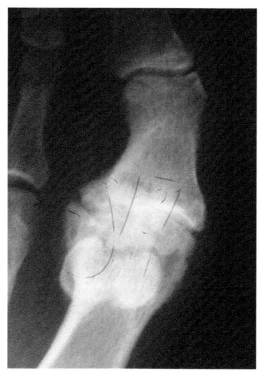

Fig. 2. Advanced OA of the first MTP.

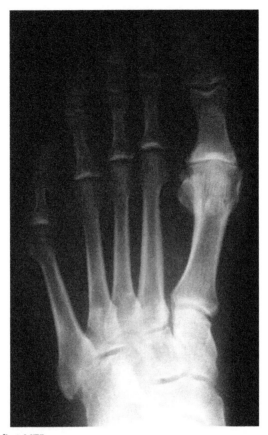

Fig. 3. OA of the first MTP.

developed a radiographic classification scheme to assess the extent of the first MTP degeneration. This classification system consists of 3 grades (**Table 1**). Coughlin and Shurnas[8] developed a grading system based on the range of motion of the first MTP, radiographic findings, and clinical presentation (**Table 2**). Other studies have proposed radiographic classifications as well.[27,28] It is thought that the more advanced the disease, the poorer the surgical outcome. Several investigators have correlated the degree of radiographic changes to surgical outcome, making the classifications somewhat of a prognostic indicator.[28–30]

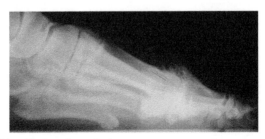

Fig. 4. First MTP OA with dorsal exostosis.

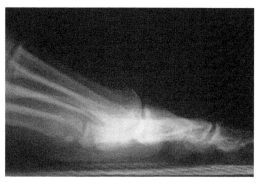

Fig. 5. Hallux rigidus grade 1.

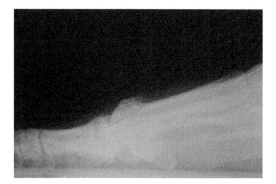

Fig. 6. Hallux rigidus grade 2.

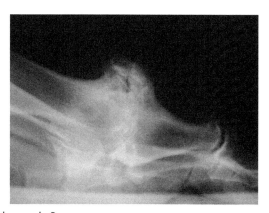

Fig. 7. Hallux rigidus grade 3.

Table 1 Hattrup and Johnson first MTP radiographic classification	
Grade 1	Mild to moderate osteophyte formation but good joint space preservation
Grade 2	Moderate osteophyte formation with joint space narrowing and subchondral sclerosis
Grade 3	Marked osteophyte formation and loss of visible joint space, with or without subchondral cyst formation

Data from Hattrup SJ, Johnson KA. Subjective results of hallux rigidus following treatment with cheilectomy. Clin Orthop Relat Res 1988;226:184.

NONOPERATIVE TREATMENT

Nonoperative treatments for hallux rigidus focus on restricting first MTP motion to decrease dorsal impingement, synovial inflammation, and pressure over dorsal osteophytes. Several nonoperative treatments for hallux rigidus have been described. The success of these treatments usually depends on the advancement of the degeneration. Activity modification, shoe wear changes, orthotics with Morton extension, NSAIDs, and injections with corticosteroid or sodium hyaluronate have been used.

The goal of orthotics and shoe wear modifications is to limit motion through the first MTP joint, thus reducing the mechanical stress on the joint.[31] Orthotics with a Morton extension effectively decreases the amount of dorsiflexion during the propulsive phase of gait and decreases symptoms. A rigid shank shoe or shoes with low heels and a rocker bottom also limit movement through the first MTP joint. Horton and colleagues[3] found that 47% of patients responded to custom orthotics alone, with another 10% responding to shoe modifications. Orthotics have been shown to provide better long-term pain relief when combined with NSAIDs than using the NSAIDs alone.[32] A wide toe box shoe is also recommended to prevent direct contact of the dorsal osteophyte with the shoe.

Corticosteroid or sodium hyaluronate injections may provide temporary relief. Patients with grade 1 OA of the first MTP reported relief for a mean of 6 months with corticosteroid injection and manipulation.[33] The same study showed a decrease in pain for 3 months in patients with grade 2 OA and no pain relief with this treatment in

Table 2 Clinical-radiographic system for grading hallux rigidus			
Grade	Dorsiflexion	Radiographs	Clinical
0	40°–60°	Normal	No pain Stiff with loss of motion
1	30°–40°	Dorsal osteophytes Minimal narrowing Minimal flattening	Mild pain and stiffness Pain with maximum DF/PF
2	10°–30°	Global osteophytes Mild/moderate narrowing	Moderate to severe pain and stiffness Relatively constant Pain near extreme ROM
3	<10°	Cystic changes	Nearly constant pain and stiffness No midrange pain
4	<10°	Same as grade 3	Grade 3 + midrange pain

Abbreviations: DF, dorsiflexion; PF, plantar flexion; ROM, range of motion.
Data from Coughlin MJ, Shurnas PS. Hallux rigidus: grading and long-term results of operative treatment. J Bone Joint Surg Am 2003;85:2072–88.

patients with grade III OA. Pons and colleagues[33] injected sodium hyaluronate into the first MTP for early stages of OA. They compared corticosteroid with sodium hyaluronate injections. The patient group with sodium hyaluronate injections had better visual analog scores and the American Orthopaedic Foot and Ankle Society (AOFAS) scores compared with the corticosteroid group. Grady and colleagues[34] reviewed 772 patients who were treated both operatively and nonoperatively for symptomatic hallux rigidus. They showed a rate of 55% success for those patients treated conservatively.

Based on the aforementioned studies, a course of conservative treatment of hallux rigidus with orthotics, shoe wear changes, or injections is successful in relieving pain of the first MTP associated with daily activities. A trial on the nonoperative treatment of symptomatic hallux rigidus patients should be considered before surgical intervention.

OPERATIVE TREATMENT

Surgical treatments of hallux rigidus have been described by various clinicians and include numerous techniques. These techniques are made up of 2 broad categories: joint salvage and joint destructive techniques. Joint salvage techniques include cheilectomy, metatarsal osteotomies, and phalangeal osteotomies. Joint destructive techniques include arthrodesis, resection arthroplasty, interpositional arthroplasty, and implant arthroplasty. Several factors including age, activity level, and severity of the disease are weighed when choosing the most appropriate surgical technique. Individual patient demands and expectation are important considerations when surgical intervention is warranted.

CHEILECTOMY

Since the original description of hallux rigidus by Davies-Colley[1] in 1887, physicians have been seeking various options for effective treatment of this condition. Cheilectomy is a common technique that entails the excision of an irregular osseous rim that interferes with motion of the joint. Cheilectomy has been described by numerous investigators as the resection of 20% to 30% of the articular surface of the dorsal aspect of the first metatarsal head.[8,35,36] The technique for cheilectomy was originally described by DuVries[6] in 1959 and reported by Mann in 1979.[37] The arthroplasty is generally made from dorsal proximal to distal plantar while maintaining a perpendicular angle to the long axis of the first metatarsal. The indications for cheilectomy described in the literature have varied greatly.[8,35,36] Much debate remains for the use of cheilectomy in moderate to severe stages of hallux rigidus. Coughlin and Shurnas support the use of the cheilectomy for all levels of disease except grade 4.

Mann and Clanton[38] treated 28 patients with 34 cheilectomies and achieved acceptable results. The average length of follow-up was 56 months. The preoperative arc of motion of the first MTP joint averaged 29°. They considered 100° as the normal arc, which was composed of 70° of dorsiflexion and 30° of plantar flexion. Dorsiflexion was limited to 30° or less in all but 2 patients.[8] The range of motion of the first MTP joint improved after cheilectomy in 23 of 31 feet. The average postoperative arc of motion was 48°, which was approximately 20° of improvement.[8] About 30° or more of dorsiflexion was achieved in 21 feet.[8]

The incision for the cheilectomy is made from distal to proximal on the dorsal aspect of the first MTP joint, just medial to the extensor hallucis longus tendon (**Fig. 8**). Capsular incision quickly exposes the arthritic joint with its associated exostosis, synovitis, and possible loose bodies (**Fig. 9**). With a 6-mm straight osteotome, an aggressive osteotomy of the dorsal exostosis is performed from distal to proximal to prevent fragmentation of the articular surface (**Fig. 10**). Advances in technology

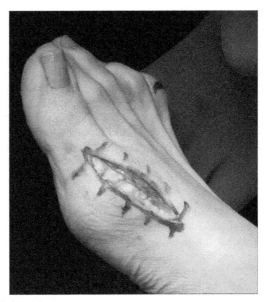

Fig. 8. Dorsal medial incision.

have led to most surgeons using power instrumentation for the osteotomy. After the osteotomy, the joint typically is passively dorsiflexed to approximately 70° without impingement.[8] Capsular and skin closure is then achieved.[8] Patients were instructed to immediately practice weight bearing with a surgical shoe.

Cheilectomy has been shown to eliminate the impingement of the first MTP joint and permits additional dorsiflexion. If further deterioration of the joint occurs, cheilectomy permits the later use of an additional procedure. This advantage does not always apply for the other procedures mentioned previously.

One of the primary issues with hallux rigidus is the recurrence of chondrolysis and exostosis following operative treatment. Easley and colleagues[39] reported that dorsal osteophytes recurred in 21 of 68 feet following cheilectomy. The investigators did not specify how this was quantified. Several others have noted that the MTP joint deteriorates radiographically following cheilectomy.[8,35,36] Smith and colleagues[31] reported

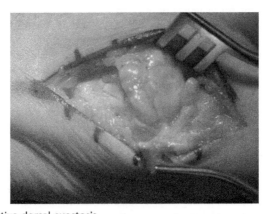

Fig. 9. Intraoperative dorsal exostosis.

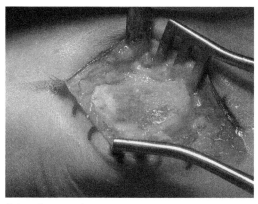

Fig. 10. Resection of dorsal exostosis.

on the natural history of hallux rigidus treated nonoperatively and observed that deterioration occurred clinically and radiographically in 16 of 24 feet. Cheilectomy does not seem to alter the degeneration process but enables patients to be more comfortable during the natural progression of the disease.[8] Cheilectomy in general is considered a temporary relief from the pain associated with the degenerative process. However, as many studies have shown, the length of pain relief is typically measured in years.[40]

Relief of pain following cheilectomy has been reported consistently, but some investigators have noted less pain relief in more advanced stages of the disease.[8,35] There is a certain point at which the cheilectomy becomes less predictable in later stages of hallux rigidus. Easley and colleagues[39] reported pain at mid range of motion in grade 4 hallux rigidus following cheilectomy. Mann and Clanton[38] reported that 22 of 25 patients treated by cheilectomy had adequate or complete relief of pain. The results of these studies indicate that cheilectomy effectively reduces pain in the treatment of hallux rigidus.

IMPLANT ARTHROPLASTY

Implant arthroplasty has been used as an alternative procedure to treat hallux rigidus over the past 60 years. There are mixed results on the efficacy and long-term results of the use of implant arthroplasty for the treatment of hallux rigidus.[8,35,36,41,42] The benefits of implant arthroplasty include decreased pain and mobility of the first MTP joint. The complications of implant arthroplasty include pain, osteolysis, transfer metatarsalgia, foreign body reaction, and late failure of the device. The primary goal of implant arthroplasty is to relieve pain and restore normal joint function to the first MTP joint. A comprehensive review of the literature may help to better understand the use and effectiveness of implant arthroplasty in the treatment of hallux rigidus.

First MTP joint implants were first introduced in the early 1950s. The first design was made from bone cement and acrylic methacrylate by Endler[43] in 1951. The basic concept of the design was to recreate the base of the proximal phalanx. The next series of implants were those of metal, which were designed to recreate the head of the first metatarsal. In 1952, Swanson[44] designed a metal hemispherical cap with a metal stem as a substitute for the first metatarsal head. The implant was deemed unsuccessful because of the rigidity of the implant.[44,45] In 1964, Seeburger[46] designed a series of implants to make a first metatarsal head prosthesis. The first design was composed of duralumin with a double flange design to fasten to the first metatarsal head with 2 self-tapping screws.[44,45,47] These implants were designed to correct patients with moderate to severe hallux valgus deformity. Several other hemiarthroplasty implants were constructed during the 1960s without much success.

The next series of advancements came in 1965, when Swanson adapted his first design to include the use of silicone. The Silastic great toe implant was a single-stemmed implant, with a silicone cap designed to replace the base of the proximal phalanx. The implant was used in conjunction with the Keller arthroplasty by acting as a spacer to maintain the normal weight-bearing property of the first MTP joint.[44,45,48] The spacer allowed for the soft tissues surrounding the joint to stabilize the motion created by the Keller arthroplasty.

Early designs proved to be inadequate for the treatment of hallux rigidus. Ris and colleagues[49] reported on 53 patients who had 68 Silastic hinged implants of the Swanson design after an average of 48 months. Physical examination of the patients revealed a decrease in the range of motion of the first MTP joint.[50] Mechanical failure of the implant, described as either fracture of the implant or permanent deformation, was noted in 57% of the patients on radiographic examination.[50]

In the early 1980s, adaptations to the implant design improved its effectiveness. Sutter created 2 Silastic double-stemmed hinged implants. The first, the Lawrence design, featured a Silastic stem angulated 15° in the sagittal plane to correspond with the normal metatarsal declination angle.[50,51] The phalangeal portion of the Lawrence design was engineered to accommodate the flexor hallucis brevis tendon to maintain its normal insertion into the base of the proximal phalanx. This modification allowed the flexor hallucis brevis to operate at full strength along with normal sesamoid function.[50,52] The LaPorta design is similar to the Lawrence design, with the addition of broad collars to prevent the bone surfaces from cutting into the implant at the base of the proximal phalanx and the head of the first metatarsal.[53] The LaPorta implant also has a 10° stem angulation built into the implant to provide physicians with the option of left, right, and neutral implants.[51] The mechanics of the designs of Sutter and Swanson differ in their approaches to achieving dorsiflexion. Swanson relied on the viscoelastic properties of the silicone, whereas Sutter allowed the hinge portion to attain dorsiflexion.[50]

Multiple studies were conducted to gauge the efficacy of flexible hinged implants. Granberry and colleagues[50] conducted a retrospective study on 90 consecutive flexible hinged implants after a 3-year follow-up period. Subjectively, most patients achieved satisfactory results with respect to pain, which was the most common preoperative symptom. However, the frequency of failure was directly correlated to the length of time the implant was in place. Granberry and colleagues[50] found 3 major faults in the use of flexible hinged implants. On examination, 30% of the patients achieved less than 15° of plantar flexion. Plantar flexion of the hallux is a key component necessary for normal propulsion during the gait cycle. The second complication of the implant is the occurrence of lesions noted to the plantar aspect of the lesser metatarsals. Painful plantar keratoses were noted beneath one metatarsal heads in 69% of the patients,[36,50] a result of shortening of the first MTP joint. Osteophyte formation at or around the first MTP joint was the third complication noted by Granberry and colleagues. Radiographic examination revealed osteophyte formation around the implant in 53% of patients.

In addition, Kampner[54] reviewed the use of the Sutter implant and reported excellent or good results in 69% of patients, in whom normal plantar flexion of the hallux was noted on physical examination.[54] The incidence of fracture of the implant was 9% at an average of 7.4 years follow-up.[54] Although subjectively patients showed good results, objectively, Silastic hinged implants did not restore normal joint function and lacked durability.

Third-Generation Implants

Decades of research and technological advances led to the third-generation first metatarsal joint implants. Third-generation Silastic implants feature more advanced materials and are designed through the use of computerized systems to consider the dynamic and static joint-specific anatomy. These designs proved to be longer lasting and more durable than first- and second-generation implants.[35,36,50] Futura Biomedical (San Diego, CA, USA) has made significant contributions to third-generation implants. In 1997, they introduced a flexible implant that featured a silicone elastomer that advanced physical properties in critical areas of tensile strength and tear resistance. Futura also designed the original third-generation, double-stemmed implant for the first MTP joint. The use of computers demonstrated that all second-generation, double-stemmed implants had one major flaw in design.[8] Second-generation designs were modeled after hand implants. Hand-implant designs featured the face and the stem of the implant coming off the hinge opposite each other. The concept of this design was to have the metatarsal head and the base of the phalanx purchase the ground during weight bearing. Designers did not take into consideration the metatarsal head, which rests on the sesamoid complex and elevates the metatarsal head in respect to the phalangeal base.[8] This flaw led to increased stress on the implant device. Third-generation, double-stemmed implants compensate for the angular disparity between the metatarsal head and the base of the proximal phalanx.

Third-generation implants were manufactured using a metallic material–designed press fit as either hemi or total implants. One of the most popular of these designs was the Biomet Total Toe System (Biomet, Warsaw, IN, USA), also known as the Koenig. Introduced in 1988, the Koenig total great toe implant is a 2-component, press-fitted implant not requiring bone cement. The first metatarsal head component comprised titanium alloy, whereas the phalangeal component comprised ultrahigh-molecular-weight polyethylene (UHMWPE), originally used in hip and knee replacements. Newer designs of this implant feature the metatarsal head comprising a cobalt-chrome cap with titanium plasma–sprayed stem. The cobalt-chrome cap provides for enhanced wear protection against the UHMWPE portion of the phalangeal base. The titanium-sprayed stem and articular surfaces of the metatarsal component provide enhanced osteointegration into the medullary canal.

Koenig devised a scoring system to evaluate the results of the Biomet Total Toe System. The scoring system was based on the Harris hip score. The scoring system was divided into 4 main categories: pain, function, range of motion, and radiographic evaluation. The scoring system is based on an overall 100-point scale. The Koenig score was used in 61 cases using the Biomet Total Toe System over a 60-month period. Of the 61 cases, 51 reported excellent results.[55–58] The average preoperative Koenig score was 31.7, and the average postoperative score was 88.[58] Based on the scoring system, 83.5% of the cases reviewed showed excellent results.[58] However, independent studies with long-term follow-up for Biomet Total Toe system are limited.

Another third-generation implant, the BioAction Great Toe (OsteoMed, Addison, TX, USA) features a metatarsal component constructed of cobalt-chrome, with a phalangeal base component constructed of titanium and polypropylene. The stems of the implant are designed to fit into the medullary canals of both the first metatarsal and the proximal phalanx. Pulavarti and colleagues[59] reported a 77% satisfaction rate, whereas the other 33% showed radiographic evidence of loosening and subsidence. The 77% satisfaction rate is poor compared with arthrodesis of the first MTP joint, which is considered by many as the procedure of choice for severe hallux rigidus.[8,35,36] Brodsky and colleagues[60] performed arthrodesis of 60 feet in 53 patients and reported a 94% satisfaction, a 100% union rate, and effective pain relief.

Similarly, the BioPro first MTP hemiarthroplasty implant (BioPro, Port Huron, MI, USA) was first introduced in 1952 by Townley and Taranow.[42] The BioPro implant is a metallic hemi-implant composed of cobalt-chrome with a press-fit tapered stem. Townley and Taranow reported 93% good or excellent results on 279 implants with an 8-month to 33-year follow-up.[42] They investigators concluded that, compared with earlier prosthesis, the BioPro implant is less likely to loosen and results in less bone loss.[42] Raikin and colleagues[36] reported on 21 hemiarthroplasties and 27 arthrodesis on 46 patients. He reported that 24% of the hemiarthroplasties failed, 1 was revised, and 4 were converted to arthrodesis. The mean follow-up of this study was 79.4 months. The mean pain score was 2.4 of 10 for hemiarthroplasty and 0.7 of 10 for the arthrodesis group. He reported that one advantage of the BioPro implant over first-generation implants was that less bone resection was required for implantation of the device.[36] Although Townley and Taranow reported good or excellent results in 93% of patients, we are not aware of any independent studies with long-term results.

Another example is the ReFlexion prosthesis (OsteoMed). This design consists of 3 components: a metatarsal stem, a phalangeal stem, and a metatarsal head. All components are interchangeable and available in 3 sizes. Based on the quality of the cancellous bone, the components can be inserted with or without bone cement.[52] Because the surgical technique is guided by an appropriate instrumentation device to facilitate positioning of the implants, the release of the plantar capsule, including a debridement of the sesamoids, seems to be more demanding.[52] Data collected from the prospective study showed (follow-up 39 months) encouraging results for pain relief and range of motion. According to the score of the AOFAS, the results improved from 51 points preoperatively to 74 points postoperatively.[52] Radiographic examination revealed radiolucent lines in 25% of the phalangeal components and in 10% of the metatarsal components. These findings were mainly attributed to a cemented fixation technique and did not impair the clinical results.[52] Like many of the previously discussed implants, the subjective results have shown success. More objective studies with long-term results should be collected to obtain further information regarding the efficacy of the ReFlexion implant in patients with hallux rigidus.

The newest first hemi-implant on the market is the Movement Great Toe System (Ascension Orthopedics, Austin, TX, USA). The anatomically shaped first MTP joint implant features a cobalt-chrome articular surface with a titanium plasma spray on the backside for enhanced osteointegration. The stem of the Movement differs from most current designs on the market. The cylindrical 4-fin stem offers press-fit fixation and antirotation stability. The metatarsal implant features a dorsal flange to prevent against recurrent osteophyte formation. The proximal phalanx component contains suture holes on the plantar portion of the implant to allow for reattachment of the flexor apparatus if compromised. The implant is available in 4 sizes and uses a conical reaming approach for minimal bone resection and retention of plantar soft tissue structures. The Movement Great Toe was first implanted on January 29, 2010, by Montross. Because of the recent introduction of the Movement Great Toe System to the market, there are no long-term studies available.

ARTHRODESIS

Arthrodesis is considered the gold standard for end-stage OA of the first MTP joint.[8,61–63] Clutton[61] first described the procedure in 1894 for hallux valgus treatment. It is a highly successful and acceptable option for patients who have advanced-stage hallux rigidus, who are younger and more active, or who have failed previous surgical procedures. First MTP arthrodesis has also been described for severe hallux valgus and hallux varus with concomitant arthritis. The success rate of this procedure had been reported to be 77% to 100% based on preoperative diagnosis, surgical technique, and method of fixation.[64–67] Reported complications include nonunion, malunion, interphalangeal joint OA, and lateral metatarsalgia.[68,69]

Positioning of the great toe for arthrodesis is critical to the success of the procedure.[70] Many factors including metatarsus elevates, cavus foot types, and pes planus foot types should be considered when setting the position of the first MTP. Because of these variations in foot type, the floor or a flat weight-bearing surface should be used as the reference point to base the hallux alignment.[71] The advocated ideal dorsiflexion of the hallux in the sagittal plane is 30° relative to the first metatarsal or 10° to 15° to the weight-bearing surface.[65,71–76] Excessive dorsiflexion leads to less hallux purchase and dorsal irritation of the interphalangeal joint with shoe wear.[70,77] Alexander[78] stated that if the tip of the toe clears the weight-bearing surface by 4 to 8 mm then normal toe-off with limited risk of hallux overload occurs. It has been advocated to increase the amount of sagittal plane dorsiflexion in women to allow the wearing of low heels.[71,79] An ankle tourniquet or esmarch around the ankle must be used cautiously to avoid the appearance of an elevated hallux due to the tension on the extensor hallucis longus tendon.[70] Frontal plane alignment should be 0°. This position gives consideration to the toe box to avoid medial hallux irritation. Overpositioning the hallux in valgus may cause irritation of the second toe.[80] The recommendation for transverse plane alignment is 10° to 15°. Alignment by referencing the position of the nail bed of the lesser toes is an easy way to correctly position the hallux in this plane. A recent study measured postoperative hallux valgus and dorsiflexion angle radiographically to assess postoperative foot function.[81] The study showed no significant correlation between foot function and hallux position, with a median hallux valgus angle of 14° and a median dorsiflexion angle of 23°.

Once the position of the first MTP joint is determined, fixation to stabilize the joint is performed. Several forms of fixation, including chromic gut, Kirschner wires, staples, crossed screws, external fixation, and specialized plates, have been described.[65,71,74,75,82–87] Not yet described is a novel intramedullary device (HalluX, Extremity Medical, Parsippany, NJ, USA). Biomechanical strength and stiffness of different fixation methods have been tested; however, no definitive recommendations have been made.[74,84–87] Crossed screws and specialized plates have been supported extensively in the literature by favorable union rates and clinical outcomes.[65,84,88,89] In a biomechanical study, a single screw and dorsal neutralization plate demonstrated being twice as strong as 2 crossed screws.[88] This finding was also supported by Buranosky and colleagues[84] with a 6-hole dorsal plate and single lag screw. Sharma and colleagues[90] showed no statistically significant differences in time to union, union, alignment, complications, and patient satisfaction when comparing clinical and radiographic outcomes of a single screw with those of a screw and quarter tubular plate. Hyer and colleagues[91] retrospectively reviewed the use of crossed screws versus specialized plates for first MTP fusion. Again, no statistical difference was noted between the 2 groups with regard to union rates, complications, or the need for hardware removal. Rongstad and colleagues[92] compared 4 different fixation techniques, a single oblique 4-mm cancellous screw, a 4.5-mm Herbert screw, a 3/32 threaded axial pin, and a dorsal Vitallium plate. They showed the dorsal plate and Herbert screw to be the strongest, with the single 4-mm screw and Steinmann pin to have comparable strength. The element of hardware cost and fusion rate have also been studied.[83] This study compared a Herbert screw, small fragment screws, and a dorsal compression plate. With regard to cost and union rate, the small fragment screws fixation seemed to be the most favorable option.

First MTP joint exposure and joint preparation varies with surgeon preference. Skin exposure using a dorsal or medial approach has been described. Joint preparation with reamers, flat cuts, curettage, and high-speed burrs have been used for first MTP fusions.[93] There are risks and benefits with both the dorsomedial soft tissue exposure and the direct medial exposure. A dorsal incision is made just medial to the extensor hallucis longus tendon. The first MTP capsule is incised longitudinally with the skin leaving a 2- to 3-mm cuff of tissue medial to the extensor hallucis longus to aid in closure. This exposure offers a full view of the dorsal exostosis and ease of use for the conical reamer system if desired. The alternative, a medial incision, may be more cosmetically appealing. This exposure also makes the flat-cut approach to joint resection easier. Circumferential joint access is more difficult with a medial incision. The cup and cone reaming system is biomechanically more stable than the flat bone cuts.[74] Goucher and Coughlin[68] reported greater ease of use and more predictable outcomes with the cup and cone reaming system, with a 92% fusion rate. They noted that flat bone cuts require greater precision, and any change in one plane affects the other two, ultimately leading to more shortening of the first ray. The cup and cone system allows desired positioning in any plane with minimal bone shortening.

The authors' preferred method is to use a cup and cone reaming system, with fixation of either an intramedullary compression device (HalluX) or a compression screw and anatomic locking first MTP plate (**Figs. 11–14**).

The HalluX is a novel 2-component intramedullary fusion device made of titanium. In vitro studies have shown it to be 1.5 times stronger than a multiple screw construct and 3.5 times stronger than dorsal plate constructs when bending strength was tested (data from file at Extremity Medical). The HalluX also showed 2.5 times more compression than a 4.0-mm solid lag screw and 45 times more compression than a 3.5-mm dorsal plate in laboratory studies (data from file at Extremity Medical). Besides this increase in strength and resistance to bending, the intramedullary design eliminates soft tissue irritation and potential skin breakdown from the underlying plate.

After a dorsal or medial incision, based on surgeon preference, it is recommended to use the cup and cone reaming system provided for joint preparation. A 1.6-mm guidewire is placed in the center of the first metatarsal and base of the proximal phalanx with the appropriate reamer to denude the cartilage. Implants are of 3 sizes: small, 6.5 mm; medium, 7.5 mm; and large, 8.5 mm, with lengths of 30 or 40 mm. Once the appropriate size of implant is determined, the corresponding drill is advanced over

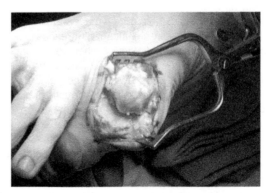

Fig. 11. First MTP access.

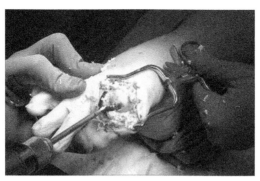

Fig. 12. Resection of metatarsal head with cup reamer.

the 1.6-mm wire into the metatarsal shaft. The implant is inserted flush with the cortical bone, leaving the window in the implant facing medial. A guidewire is then passed antegrade through the medial cortex of the first metatarsal. With the joint reduced and in position, the wire is passed retrograde across the MTP, holding the position and acting as the guidewire for the cannulated lag screw (**Fig. 15**). The lag screw is then inserted, after the correct measurement, through a dorsal window created in the bone. Compression is gained once the land of the screw interfaces and locks into the Morse taper of the metatarsal implant. Long-term data and follow-up is not yet available on this device; however, early clinical and radiographic signs are promising.

A compression lag screw with a dorsal anatomic locking plate is also the authors' preferred method of fixation. Once the joint is prepared for fusion with the cup and cone reaming system, a compression screw is inserted across the joint from distal medial to proximal lateral. A dorsal anatomic locked plate is then implanted for added strength (**Fig. 16**).

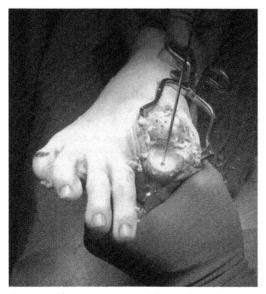

Fig. 13. Guidewire placement for cone reamer at base of proximal phalanx.

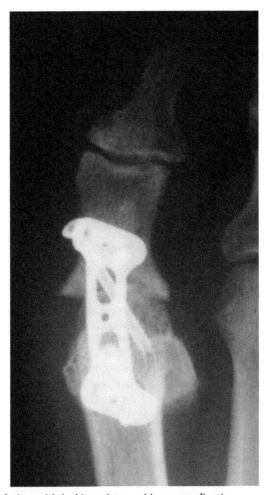

Fig. 14. First MTP fusion with locking plate and lag screw fixation.

With the advent of anatomic plates offering a more rigid construct and the inherent stability of the joint resection, early or immediate weight bearing is possible after surgery. Dayton and McCall[94] reported on immediate weight bearing postoperatively, with 18 patients in a surgical shoe. Union was noted at 6.1 weeks, with return to athletic shoes at 6.2 weeks. Hyer and colleagues[91] allowed immediate weight bearing in 37 patients with a fusion rate of 91.1%. These reports support immediate weight bearing and early return to shoe wear, thus decreasing patient morbidity postoperatively. Regardless of the joint resection technique or form of fixation, early to immediate weight bearing should be the priority for patients postoperatively.

The success of first MTP joint arthrodesis has been well documented in the literature, with high patient satisfaction rates.[23] Coughlin and Shurnas[8] reported on 34 patients who underwent arthrodesis with a mean follow-up of 6.7 years. They showed that their patients had a good or excellent result 100% of the time, with a 94% union rate and 2 asymptomatic fibrous unions. No hallux interphalangeal joint arthrosis was reported. Raikin and colleagues[36] compared first MTP arthrodesis to metallic

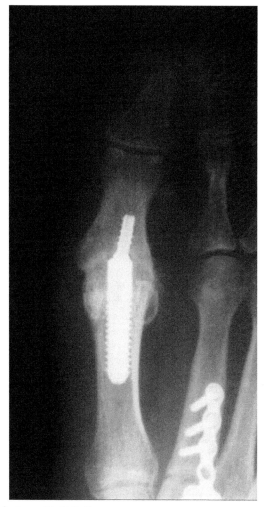

Fig. 15. First MTP fusion with HalluX.

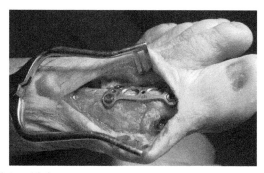

Fig. 16. Locking plate with lag screw.

hemiarthroplasty. They showed a statistically significant better satisfaction rate at a mean follow-up of 79.4 months in the fusion group. Goucher and Coughlin[68] reported on 49 patients who underwent first MTP fusion with a minimum of 1 year of follow-up. The fusion rate was 92%, and patient satisfaction was 96%, with improvement in pain and AOFAS scores. A 100% fusion rate and improvement in AOFAS and short form-36 (SF-36) scores were reported by Flavin and Stephens.[95] Twenty patients underwent first MTP arthrodesis for a variety of preoperative diagnoses. The average follow-up in this study was 18 months.

First MTP joint arthrodesis for end-stage hallux rigidus, failed previous surgical intervention, and severe hallux valgus of OA has been show to be both predictable and reproducible with good to excellent results. Biomechanically, no disability or adverse affect on gait has been noted, and this procedure restores the weight-bearing function of the first ray, reducing transfer metatarsalgia.

SUMMARY

Comparing various operations for the treatment of hallux rigidus is a difficult task. In patients seeking an alternative to arthrodesis, implant arthroplasty and cheilectomy offer a reduction in pain and increased mobility. Each procedure has its own unique indications and ideal patient populations. Implant arthroplasty has gone through significant changes over the past 6 decades, with advancements in technology facilitating dramatic changes in materials and surgical technique. Newer-generation implants feature a more durable construction with less bone resection during implantation. These advancements have resulted in higher patient satisfaction with a longer implant life. Because fourth-generation implants do not have long-term data, third-generation implants should provide insight for future consideration in implant design and long-term outcome.

Third-generation implants have shown good or excellent results subjectively in patients. They offer relief of pain and increased mobility of the first MTP joint. Objective examination and long-term durability of the implants have not been as favorable. Fracture and deformation of the implants over a long period is a complication commonly seen in implant arthroplasty. Recurrence and osteolysis are also common complications that should be considered when using implants for the treatment of hallux rigidus. Although significant advancements have been made in implant arthroplasty, cheilectomy and arthrodesis is a more predictable procedure that offers greater patient satisfaction over a longer period. Cheilectomy offers decreased pain and increased mobility with fewer complications than first MTP joint implants. In regards to treatment of hallux rigidus, surgical intervention should result in decreased pain, increased range of motion, and long-term durability.

REFERENCES

1. Davies-Colley M. Contraction of the metatarso-phalangeal joint of the great toe. BMJ 1887;1:728.
2. Cotterill J. Stiffness of the great toe in adolescents. BMJ 1888;1:1158.
3. Horton GA, Park YW, Myerson MS. Role of metatarsus primus elevattus in the pathogenesis of hallux rigidus. Foot Ankle Int 1999;20(12):777–80.
4. Van Saase JL, Van Romunde LK, Cats A, et al. Epidemiology of osteoarthritis: Zoetermeer survey. Comparison of radiological osteoarthritis in a Dutch population with that in 10 other population. Ann Rheum Dis 1989;48:271–80.
5. Nilsonne H. Hallux rigidus and its treatment. Acta Orthop Scand 1930;1:295–302.

6. DuVries H. Static deformities. In: DuVries H, editor. Surgery of the foot. St Louis (MO): Mosby; 1959. p. 392–8.
7. Moberg E. A simple operation for hallux rigidus. Clin Orthop Relat Res 1979;142: 55–6.
8. Coughlin MJ, Shurnas PS. Hallux rigidus: grading and long-term results of operative treatment. J Bone Joint Surg Am 2003;85(11):2072–88.
9. Anderson W. Lectures on contractions of the fingers and toes; their varieties, pathology and treatment. Lancet 1891;138:279–82. Available at: http://dx.doi. org/10.1016.s0140-736(02)01248-5. Accessed August, 2010.
10. Bonney G, Macnab I. Hallux valgus and hallux rigidus; a critical survey of operative results. J Bone Joint Surg Br 1952;34:366–85.
11. Bingold AC, Collins DH. Hallux rigidus. J Bone Joint Surg Br 1950;32:214–22.
12. Shrader JA, Siegel KL. Nonoperative management of functional hallux limitus in a patient with rheumatoid arthritis. Phys Ther 2003;83:831–43.
13. Jack EA. The aetiology of hallux rigidus. Br J Surg 1940;27:492–7.
14. Cicchinelli LD, Casmasta CA, McGlamry ED. Latrogenic metatarsus primus elevates. Etiology, evaluation and surgical management. J Am Podiatr Med Assoc 1997;87:165–77.
15. McMurray TP. Treatment of hallux valgus and rigidus. Br Med J 1936;2:218–21.
16. Sim-Fook L, Hodgson AR. A comparison of foot forms among the non-shoe and shoe-wearing Chinese population. J Bone Joint Surg Am 1958;40:1058–62.
17. Lambrinudi P. Metatarsus primus elevatus. Proc R Soc Med 1938;31:1273.
18. Meyer JO, Nishon JR, Weiss L, et al. Metatarsus primus elevates and the etiology of hallux rigidus. J Foot Surg 1987;26:237–41.
19. Mahiquez MY, Wilder FV, Stephens HM. Positive hindfoot valgus and osteoarthritis of the first metatarsophalangeal joint. Foot Ankle Int 2006;27(12):1055–9.
20. Zammit GV, Menz HB, Munteanu SE. Structural factors associated with hallux limitus/rigidus: a systematic review of case control studies. J Orthop Sports Phys Ther 2009;39(10):733–42.
21. Coughlin MJ, Shurnas PS. Hallux rigidus: demographics, etiology and radiographic assessment. Foot Ankle Int 2003;3(24):731–43.
22. Coughlin MJ. Conditions of the forefoot. In: DeLee J, Drez D, editors. Orthopaedic sports medicine: principles and practice. Philadelphia: WB Saunders; 1994. p. 221–444.
23. Yee G, Lau J. Current concepts review: hallux rigidus. Foot Ankle Int 2008;29(6): 637–46.
24. Lapidus PW. Dorsal bunion: its mechanics and operative correction. J Bone Joint Surg 1940;22:627–37.
25. Beeson P, Phillips C, Corr S, et al. Classification systems for hallux rigidus: a review of the literature. Foot Ankle Int 2008;29(4):407–14.
26. Hattrup SJ, Johnson KA. Subjective results of hallux rigidus following treatment with cheilectomy. Clin Orthop Relat Res 1988;226:182–91.
27. Regnauld B. The foot: pathology, aetiology, seminology, clinical investigation and treatment. New York: Springer-Verlag; 1986.
28. Hanft JR, Mason ET, Landsman AS, et al. A new radiographic classification for hallux limitus. J Foot Ankle Surg 1993;32:397–404.
29. Geldwert JJ, Rock GD, McGrath MP, et al. Cheilectomy: still a useful technique for grade I and grade II hallux limitus/rigidus. J Foot Surg 1992;31:154–9.
30. Pontell D, Gudas CJ. Retrospective analysis of surgical treatment of hallux rigidus/limitus: clinical and radiographic follow-up of hinged, silastic implant arthroplasty and cheilectomy. J Foot Surg 1988;27:503–10.

31. Smith RW, Katchis SD, Ayson LC. Outcomes in hallux rigidus patients treated nonoperatively: a long-term follow-up study. Foot Ankle Int 2000;21(11):906–13.
32. Thompson JA, Jennings MB, Hodge W. Orthotic therapy in the management of osteoarthritis. J Am Podiatr Med Assoc 1992;82:136–9.
33. Pons M, Alvarez F, Solana J, et al. Sodium hyaluronate in the treatment of hallux rigidus. A single blind, randomized study. Foot Ankle Int 2007;28(1):38–42.
34. Grady JF, Axe TM, Zager EJ, et al. A retrospective analysis of 772 patients with hallux limitus. J Am Podiatr Med Assoc 2002;92(2):102–8.
35. Beeson P. The surgical treatment of hallux limitus/rigidus: a critical review of the literature. Foot 2004;14:6–22.
36. Raikin SM, Ahmad J, Pour AE, et al. Comparison of arthrodesis and metallic hemi-arthroplasty of the hallux metatarsophalangeal joint. J Bone Joint Surg Am 2007; 89(9):1979–85.
37. Mann RA, Coughlin MJ, DuVries HL. Hallux Rigidus: a review of the literature and a method of treatment. Clin Orthop Relat Res 1979;142:57–63.
38. Mann RA, Clanton TO. Hallux rigidus: treatment by cheilectomy. J Bone Joint Surg Am 1988;70(3):400–6.
39. Easley ME, Davis WH, Anderson RB. Intermediate to long-term follow-up of medial-approach dorsal cheilectomy for hallux rigidus. Foot Ankle Int 1999; 20(3):147–52.
40. Bussewitz BW, Dyment M, Hyer CF. Intermediate-term results following first meta-tarsal cheilectomy. Poster presentation at the 2011 American College of Foot and Ankle Surgeons Annual Scientific Meeting. Ft Lauderdale (FL), March 9–12, 2011.
41. Giannini S, Moroni A. Alumina total joint replacement of the first metatarsophalan-geal joint. In: Bonfield W, Hastings GW, Tanner KE, editors. Bioceramics, vol 4. London: Butterworth-Heineman; 1991. p. 39–45.
42. Townley CO, Taranow WS. A metallic hemiarthroplasty resurfacing prosthesis for the hallux metatarsophalangeal joint. Foot Ankle Int 1994;15(11):575–80.
43. Endler F. Zur entwicklung einer kuenstilichen arthro -plasik des grosszenhen-grudgel enke unde ihrebisheride indekation. Z Orthop Grenzgeb 1951;80(3): 480–7 [in German].
44. Swanson AB. Implant arthroplasty for the great toe. Clin Orthop Relat Res 1972; 85:75–81.
45. Swanson AB, de Groot Swanson G. Use of grommets for flexible hinge implant arthroplasty of the great toe. Clin Orthop Relat Res 1997;340:87–94.
46. Seeburger RH. Surgical implants of alloyed metal injoints of the feet. J Am Podi-atry Assoc 1964;54:391.
47. Hetherington V, Cwikla P, Malone M, editors. Textbook of hallux valgus and fore-foot surgery. 2000.
48. Swanson AB, Lumsden RM, Swanson GD. Silicone implant arthroplasty of the great toe. A review of single stem and flexible hinge implants. Clin Orthop Relat Res 1979;142:30–43.
49. Ris HB, Mettler M, Engeloch F. Langzeitergebnisse mit der Silastik-Endoprothese nach Swanson am Grosszehengrundgelenk. Diskrepanz zwischen Klinik und radiologischem Befund. Z Orthop Grenzgeb 1988;126(5):526–9 [in German].
50. Granberry WM, Noble PC, Bishop JO, et al. Use of a hinged silicone prosthesis for replacement arthroplasty of the first metatarsophalangeal joint. J Bone Joint Surg Am 1991;73(10):1453–9.
51. Jarvis BD, Moats DB, Burns A, et al. Lawrence design first metatarsophalangeal joint prosthesis. J Am Podiatr Med Assoc 1986;76:617.

52. Lawrence BR, Papier MJ 2nd. Implant arthroplasty of the lesser metatarsophalangeal joint—a modified technique. J Foot Surg 1980;19(1):16–8.
53. LaPorta GA, Pilla P Jr, Richter KP. Keller implant procedure: a report of 536 procedures using a Silastic intramedullary stemmed implant. J Am Podiatry Assoc 1976;66(3):126–47.
54. Kampner SL. Long-term experience with total joint prosthetic replacement for the arthritic great toe. Bull Hosp Jt Dis Orthop Inst 1987;47(2):153–77.
55. Koenig RD. Koenig total great toe implant. Preliminary report. J Am Podiatr Med Assoc 1990;80(9):462–8.
56. Koenig RD. Revision arthroplasty utilizing the Biomet Total Toe System for failed silicone elastomer implants. J Foot Ankle Surg 1994;33(3):222–7.
57. Koenig RD. Total toe implant. 2008. Available at: http://www.greattoe.com/. Accessed August, 2010.
58. Koenig RD, Horwitz LR. The Biomet Total Toe System utilizing the Koenig score: a five-year review. J Foot Ankle Surg 1996;35(1):23–6.
59. Pulavarti RS, McVie JL, Tulloch CJ. First metatarsophalangeal joint replacement using the bio-action great toe implant: intermediate results. Foot Ankle Int 2005;26(12):1033–7.
60. Brodsky JW, Ptaszek AJ, Morris SG. Salvage first MTP arthrodesis utilizing ICBG: clinical evaluation and outcome. Foot Ankle Int 2000;21(4):290–6.
61. Clutton HH. The treatment of hallux valgus. St Thomas Rep 1894;22:1–12.
62. Sheriff MJ, Baumhauer JF. Hallux rigidus and osteoarthrosis of the first metatarsophalangeal joint. J Bone Joint Surg Am 1998;80(6):898–908.
63. Lombardi CM, Silhanek AD, Connolly FG, et al. First metatarsophalangeal arthrodesis for treatment of hallux rigidus: a retrospective study. J Foot Ankle Surg 2001;40(3):137–43.
64. Coughlin MJ. Arthrodesis of the first metatarsophalangeal joint with mini-fragment plate fixation. Orthopedics 1990;13:1037–44.
65. Coughlin MJ, Abdo RV. Arthrodesis of the first metatarsophalangeal joint with Vitallium plate fixation. Foot Ankle Int 1994;15:18–28.
66. Gimple K, Anspacher J, Kopta J. Metatarsophalangeal joint fusion of the great toe. Orthopedics 1978;1:462–7.
67. Von Salis-Soglio G, Thomas W. Arthrodesis of the metatarsophalangeal joint of the great toe. Arch Orthop Trauma Surg 1979;95:7–12.
68. Goucher NR, Coughlin MJ. Hallux metatarsophalangeal joint arthrodesis using dome-shaped reamers and dorsal plate fixation: a prospective study. Foot Ankle Int 2006;27(11):869–76.
69. Keller WL. The surgical treatment of bunions and hallux valgus. New York Med J 1904;80:741–2.
70. Womack JW, Ishikawa SN. First metatarsophalangeal arthrodesis. Foot Ankle Clin 2009;14:43–50.
71. Kelikian AS. Technical considerations in hallux metatarsophalangeal arthrodesis. Foot Ankle Clin 2005;10:167–90.
72. Bouché RT, Adad JM. Arthrodesis of the first metatarsaophalangeal joint in active people. Clin Podiatr Med Surg 1996;13(3):461–84.
73. Wu KK. First metatarsophalangeal fusion in the salvage of failed hallux abducto valgus operations. J Foot Ankle Surg 1994;33(4):383–95.
74. Curtis MJ, Myerson M, Jinnah RH, et al. Arthrodesis of the first metatarsophalangeal joint: a biomechanical study of internal fixation techniques. Foot Ankle 1993;14(7):395–9.

75. Riggs SA, Johnson EW, McKeever D. Arthrodesis for the painful hallux. Foot Ankle 1983;3:248–53.
76. Fitzgerald JA, Wilkinson JM. Arthrodesisof the metatarsophalangeal joint of the great toe. Clin Orthop Relat Res 1981;157:70–7.
77. Hamilton GA, Ford LA, Patel S. First metatarsophalangeal joint arthrodesis and revision arthrodesis. Clin Podiatr Med Surg 2009;26:459–73.
78. Alexander IJ. Hallux metatarsophalangeal joint arthrodesis. In: Kitakoa HB, editor. Masters techniques in foot and ankle surgery. 2nd edition. Philadelphia: Lippincott Williams and Wilkins; 2002. p. 45–60.
79. Esway JE, Conti SF. Joint replacement in the hallux metatarsophalangeal joint. Foot Ankle Clin 2005;10(10):97–115.
80. Fitzgerald JAW. A review of long-term results of first metatarsophalangeal arthrodesis. J Bone Joint Surg Br 1969;51:488–93.
81. Van doeselaar DJ, Heesterbeek PJC, Louwerens JWK, et al. Foot function after fusion of the first metatarsophalangeal joint. Foot Ankle Int 2010;31(8):670–5.
82. O'Doherty DP, Lowrie IG, Magnussen PA, et al. The management of painful first metatarsophalangeal joint in the older patient: arthrodesis or Keller arthroplasty? J Bone Joint Surg Br 1990;72:839–42.
83. Watson AD, Kelikian AS. Cost effectiveness comparison of three methods of internal fixation for arthrodesis of the first metatarsophalangeal joint. Foot Ankle Int 1988;19(5):304–10.
84. Buranosky DJ, Taylor DT, Sage RA, et al. First metatarsophalangeal joint arthrodesis: quantitative mechanical testing of six hole dorsal plate versus crossed screw fixation in cadaveric specimens. J Foot Ankle Surg 2001;40(4): 208–13.
85. Molloy S, Burkhart BG, Jasper BS, et al. Biomechanical comparison of two fixation methods for first metatarsophalangeal joint arthrodesis. Foot Ankle Int 2001;24(2):169–71.
86. Neufeld SK, Parks BG, Naseef GS, et al. Arthrodesis of the first metatarsophalangeal joint: a biomechanical study comparing memory compression staples, cannulated screws and a dorsal plate. Foot Ankle Int 2002;23(2):97–101.
87. Sage RA, Lam AT, Taylor DT. Retrospective analysis of first metatarsophalangeal joint arthrodesis. J Foot Ankle Surg 1997;36:425–9.
88. Politi J, John H, Njus G, et al. First metatarsal-phalangeal joint arthrodesis: a biomechanical assessment of stability. Foot Ankle Int 2003;24(4):332–7.
89. Swiatek M, Ringus VM, Hyer CF. A retrospective comparison of four plate constructs for first metatarsophalangeal joint fusion: static plate, static plate with lag screw, locked plate, locked plate with lag screw. Poster presentation at the 2010 American College of Foot and Ankle Surgeons (ACFAS) Annual Scientific Meeting. Las Vegas (NV), February 22–26, 2010. E-poster presentation at the 2010 American Orthopaedic Foot & Ankle Society Annual Summer Meeting. National Harbor (MD), July 7–10, 2010.
90. Sharma H, Bhagat S, Deleeuw J, et al. In vivo comparison of screw versus plate and screw fixation for first metatarsophalangeal arthrodesis: does augmentation of internal compression screw fixation using a semi-tubular plate shorten time to clinical and radiographic fusion of the first metatarsophalangeal joint (MTPJ). J Foot Ankle Surg 2008;47(1):2–7.
91. Hyer CF, Glover JP, Berlet GC, et al. Cost comparison of crossed screws versus dorsal plate construct for first metatarsophlangeal joint arthrodesis. J Foot Ankle Surg 2008;47(1):13–8.

92. Rongstad KM, Miller GJ, vadergriend RA, et al. A biomechanical comparison of four fixation methods of first metatarsophalangeal joint arthrodesis. Foot Ankle Int 1994;15:415–9.
93. Johansson JE, Barrington TW. Cone arthrodesis of the first metatarsophalangeal joint. Foot Ankle 1984;4:244–8.
94. Dayton P, McCall A. Early weightbearing after first metatarsophalangeal joint arthrodesis: a retrospective observational case analysis. J Foot Ankle Surg 2004;43(3):156–9.
95. Flavin R, Stephens MM. Arthrodesis of the first metatarsophalangeal joint using a dorsal titanium contoured plate. Foot Ankle Int 2004;25(11):783–7.

Hallux Rigidus: What Lies Beyond Fusion, Resectional Arthroplasty, and Implants

Melissa M. Galli, DPM, MHA[a], Christopher F. Hyer, DPM[b],*

KEYWORDS

• Hallux rigidus • OATS • Interpositional arthroplasty
• Arthrodiastasis

Hallux rigidus (HR) refers to the limitation of motion at the first metatarsophalangeal (MTP) joint, most commonly secondary to degenerative arthritis. Although the condition was first clinically described in 1887 by Davies-Colley as hallux flexus, the term hallux rigidus was coined by Cotterill in the same year to characterize the painful limitation of motion at the first MTP joint. Since the initial description, countless surgical variations have been described throughout the foot and ankle literature to treat this condition in adults, which is second only to hallux valgus in its prevalence at the MTP joint. HR is the most common form of osteoarthritis (OA) in the foot and ankle, with an incidence of 1 in 40 adults older than 50 years.[1]

Historically, surgical options for the treatment of HR lie in 2 general categories: joint salvage, including cheilectomy, phalangeal osteotomy, and first metatarsal osteotomy and joint destruction, which comprises excisional arthroplasty, implant arthroplasty, and arthrodesis. Over the last half-century and with increasing frequency, a hybrid of these techniques has emerged in the form of cartilage resurfacing, interpositional arthroplasty (IA), and arthrodiastasis. Theoretically, these procedures aim to address the pathologic condition of the first MTP joint more directly than joint salvage and to avoid many of the negative complications, consequences, and connotations of joint destruction procedures.

The authors have nothing to disclose.
[a] Department of Orthopaedics, The Ohio State University Medical Center, 410 West 10th Avenue, N-1050, Columbus, OH 43210, USA
[b] Orthopedic Foot and Ankle Center, 300 Polaris Parkway Suite 2000, Westerville, OH 43082, USA
* Corresponding author.
E-mail address: ofacresearch@orthofootankle.com

THE PROCEDURES AND PATIENT SELECTION

Surgical procedure preferences for the treatment of HR is similar to all avenues of elective orthopedic surgery; surgeons must synchronize between addressing the patient's pathology, balancing their expectations, and choosing a procedure in which they are well-versed and which they can execute appropriately. The literature is clear on which patients with OA of the first MTP joint need more than a cheilectomy as DuVries originally described in 1959. Pain at the mid–range of motion has been reported as a harbinger of poor postcheilectomy results by multiple investigators. In addition, advanced radiographic changes and a patient's subjective complaints should prompt a practitioner to consider an operation that addresses a joint pathologic condition in a more direct manner than a cheilectomy.[2,3] Taking away joint motion, the concept of a joint fusion or arthrodesis is often not an appealing option for many patients, particularly those who are young and active. Alternative surgical options for the treatment of recalcitrant pain associated with HR are evolving and are discussed in this review.

Every surgical option has its indications, contraindications, and relative contraindications/warnings. It is well documented that when HR is treated nonoperatively, the MTP joint deteriorates clinically with time, as observed radiographically. However, approximately 33% of patients treated with cheilectomy had dorsal osteophyte recurrence.[3] Therefore, individualizing the treatment course of HR and appropriately weighing risks and benefits of each surgical procedure are vital to patient outcomes and satisfaction.

JOINT RESURFACING

The pathophysiologic presentation of HR is intrinsically linked to OA and cartilage damage. The surgical procedures for HR address this via resection, repair, or replacement of the battered first MTP joint that is responsible to 60% to 70% of weight bearing through the propulsive phase of gait. Osteochondral lesions of the first MTP joint from a single traumatic incident or from repetitive episodes are frequently encountered surgically. In instances in which the damage is solely to the upper third of the metatarsal head, a simple cheilectomy is sufficient to remove the lesion and often reduces symptoms. For lower central lesions, resurfacing of the joint is a treatment method to more readily restore cartilage to a functional level.[4,5] This method may be performed via fibrocartilage stimulation or transfer of hyaline cartilage through an osteochondral autograft transplant system (OATS) procedure.

Fibrocartilage and Hyaline Cartilage Stimulation

The native hyaline cartilage within a joint is ideally suited for the stress and pressur within the joint. But repair or regrowth of the hyaline cartilage has proved elusive. As in other joints, marrow stimulation or abrasion arthoplasty is performed to stimulate the production of fibrocartilage in areas of hyaline cartilage damage or loss. Although fibrocartilage is non-native to the articular surface, it serves the role of a "patch" to the deficient area.

Subchondral drilling and microfracture by various instrumentation are the predominant stimulation methods. Traditionally, for the first MTP joint, stimulation has been done via open technique (**Figs. 1** and **2**). Multiple investigators, however, have advocated the use of a hallux MTP joint arthroscopy and debridement to address the pathologic condition and stimulate fibrocartilage production in young to middle-aged patients with moderate primary OA.[6,7] Although not all of the 20 patients included in this study had debridement, 95% of patients related a subjective improvement in

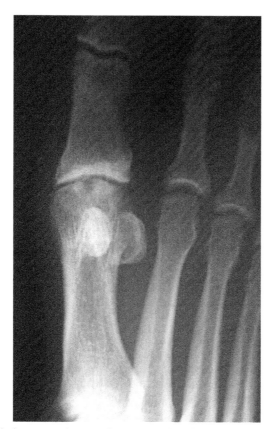

Fig. 1. Radiograph demonstrating significant osteochondral defect of first metatarsal head.

pain and swelling of the hallux MTP joint, with 90% being able to return to their former sporting activities and wear normal shoes. Mean American Orthopaedic Foot and Ankle Society (AOFAS) scores improved from 43 (10–78) preoperatively to 97 (87–100) 2 years postoperation, whereas dorsiflexion improved from an average of 8° to 30° over the same duration. Despite these positive results, resistance of stiffness and superficial sensory nerve loss were experienced in 3 patients.[7]

Hyaline cartilage regeneration is the ultimate option to improve the long-term viability of a joint, such as the hallux MTP joint, that is stricken with OA changes in HR. Ritsila and colleagues[8] observed in numerous experimental animal studies that free periosteal grafts had a tendency to favor the differentiation of cartilage in a chondrotrophic environment for which joint motion has a vital role. The investigators found that immobilization had a clearly inhibitory effect on chondrogenesis, whereas mobilization had a distinct stimulatory effect. In another study using a rabbit model, a free periosteal transplant rapidly formed cartilage tissue from periosteal cells, and this formation was strongest at 6 weeks after implantation.[9]

In 1992, this technique was used on 2 patients who had severe pain from HR for between 2 and 3.5 years. These patients were treated with periosteal resurfacing of the metatarsal head with an anterior tibial graft. The graft was sutured to the cambium layer toward the subchondral bone using resorbable polyglycolic acid suture, with the addition of fibrin glue in the second patient. At 8 and 10 years of follow-up,

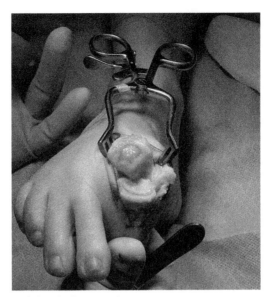

Fig. 2. Osteochondral defect before repair.

respectively, both patients were free of pain and swelling at the hallux MTP joint and had a total joint motion of 101° and 91°, respectively. The investigators recommended this treatment for young and active patients.[10] Although this research is promising, large-scale high level of evidence-based medicinal studies in humans regarding periosteal graft stimulation of hyaline cartilage at the first MTP joint are unavailable.

Hyaline Transplant via OATS

Originally used for focal osteochondritis dissecans lesions in the weight-bearing surface of the femoral condyles with promising long-term results in the knee, the OATS procedure has increasingly become an option for similar defects elsewhere in the body. The dorsal quarter to third of the metatarsal head is commonly removed by cheilectomy without sequelae. This area also serves as a possible donor site in several case reports. Also, this aspect of the metatarsal head has similar convex properties as the central portion. The OATS procedure is indicated when the defect is isolated and the dorsal cartilage of the first metatarsal head is in excellent condition.[5] This may be the case in acute injuries, but not in degenerative injuries.

Key technical considerations for an OATS procedure include a precise fit and contour matching of the graft. Instrumented guides are often used to reduce technical difficulties in matching plug sizes. This procedure and instrumentation provide an articular plug of hyaline cartilage that incorporates with surrounding tissue and restores normal biomechanics to the first MTP joint, thus reverses the present and minimizes the future joint degeneration. This potentially joint-preserving procedure can be performed alone or in combination to address concomitant pathologic conditions.[5]

Title and colleagues[5] described the following protocol for small (≤5 mm diameter) local-shift osteochondral plug transplant. A dorsal oblique cheilectomy of the proximal phalanx with a rongeur is performed to adequately expose the metatarsal head. Once the lesion is isolated, the cartilage is trimmed to healthy edges, and the size is determined with the round sizer from the OATS set (Arthrex, Naples, FL, USA). Next, the dorsal cartilage donor site is selected with care to match contour. This site is viewed with the corresponding next-size larger round sizer and is harvested to a depth of 12 mm with the aid of a mallet. Attention is then directed back to the recipient site that is harvested to 10 mm. Finally, the donor plug is tamped into the recipient site to a slight 1-mm proud position; in the literature, this elevated state is recommended to allow for some contraction of the graft as it incorporates into the surrounding tissue.[11] The MTP joint is then compressed with gentle axial loading and dorsiflexed to ensure an even gliding surface. With a chisel, metatarsal cheilectomy is then performed at the margins of the donor site, and any concomitant procedures are performed if indicated. Standard layered closure is then performed, a compressive dressing is applied, and patients are able to bear weight on their heels for the first 2 weeks, after which they may progress to activity and wear shoe gear as tolerated. For larger metatarsal head defects, successful procurement of talar and femoral articular plugs has been described (**Fig. 3**).[11–14]

Within the foot and ankle literature, 2 trauma case studies have been presented, in which well-defined radiolucent lesions are visualized with preoperative imaging.[15] In the first case study, the defect was filled with an articular graft harvested from the medial aspect of the talar head; the graft showed full incorporation 6 months postoperation on magnetic resonance imaging. Clinically, the patient had no talonavicular joint or first MTP joint pain, but did have slightly reduced dorsiflexion and plantar flexion of the latter joint in comparison to the contralateral foot.[14] In another case, a standard OATS procedure was performed with an 8-mm-diameter graft harvested from the lateral portion of the ipsilateral lateral femoral condyle. At 2 years of follow-up examination, the patient was pain free in the knee and first MTP joint, was able to obtain 50° dorsiflexion and 30° plantar flexion, and tolerated running, aerobics, and high-heeled shoe gear.[12]

Although incorporation of the transplanted plug in reported cases has been complete, there are no published reports of the rate and degree of incorporation based on graft thickness in the first MTP joint. Historically, however, these differences have not affected the long-term outcomes in OATS procedures of the talus.[11] In patients with too large a defect for local transposition and with concern over donor-site morbidity, it is important to use the allograft as a viable option, although the viability of chondrocytes and their rate and time line of incorporation remain a contentious point in the orthopedic literature. Large, multicentered, randomized controlled

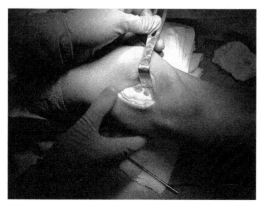

Fig. 3. Harvest site of femoral osteochondral plugs.

trials are nonexistent and desperately warranted to improve HR treatment protocols and patient outcomes with this subtype of procedures.

INTERPOSITIONAL ARTHROPLASTY

Using a biologic autograft, allograft, or xenograft soft tissue as a physical interpositional spacer in the first MTP joint addresses the shortcomings of arthrodesis and the Keller arthroplasty. Although silastic and metallic implants may do the same, patients and physicians alike may not have the same concern over the well-documented wear of these devices that are, at times, accompanied by soft tissue reactions.[15] The theoretic advantages of IA as a class of procedures include: allows less bony resection, provides greater preservation of metatarsal length, permits joint motion, and imparts joint stability with possibly a lower likelihood of foreign body reactions. Collectively, these attributes should improve subjective outcomes, overall function, and long-term success rates compared with more traditional procedures.

Hamilton and Hubbard[16] outlined the general indications of capsular IA of the first MTP joint as "a healthy, active patient with grade III symptomatic hallux rigidus or failed cheilectomy unresponsive to conservative therapy as an alternative to first (MTP) fusion." Their absolute and relative contraindications are three fold and include poor vascular status, presence of infection, or presence of neuropathy. The investigators warned against using these procedures in patients with Morton foot because a short first metatarsal has an increased risk of developing transfer metatarsalgia, in those with arthritic hallux valgus, or in those with high athletic demand because long-term results are unknown and there is concern over the implications of the windlass mechanism destruction in these populations.

Autograft: Tendocapsular Interposition

Hamilton and colleagues[1] published retrospective results of 30 patients (37 feet) with HR who were treated with capsular IA. Through a medial incision, a standard one-third cheilectomy and resection of less than 25% of the base of the proximal phalanx were performed. Next, the extensor hallucis brevis (EHB) was incised 4 cm proximal to the MTP joint. The EHB along with the joint capsule and extensor hood was then passed through the MTP joint and sutured to the flexor hallucis brevis just distal to the sesamoids (**Fig. 4**). In this study, the interphalangeal (IP) and MTP joints were then stabilized with a Kirschner (K)-wire fixation for 3 weeks. At an undisclosed period of follow-up, 28 of the 30 patients related that they were pleased with the operation and would undergo the operation again. Postoperation, there was significantly increased range of motion and radiographic joint space, whereas plantar-flexion strength remained at least 4 of 5 in all patients without complaint of a weak push-off. In a follow-up study, however, Hamilton and Hubbard[16] stated that K-wire stabilization is optional and recovery was faster without its use. They also advocated a prophylactic second metatarsal condylectomy for patients with a long second metatarsal in relation to the foot and warned that the hallux may seem "floppy" for several months postoperation because of the bony shortening until the extensor tendons shorten and active motion returns to the joint. Over the duration of the 2 studies, the investigators studied 54 patients, with 51 (94%) reporting good to excellent results.[1,16]

Kennedy and colleagues[17] and Lau and Daniels[18] reported collectively on 29 patients treated with IA of the EHB tendon and joint capsule with the Lau protocol also using K-wires across the hallux MTP and IP joints for 3 weeks. Complications included restricted motion (to <20°) in 2 patients, transfer metatarsalgia in 4 patients

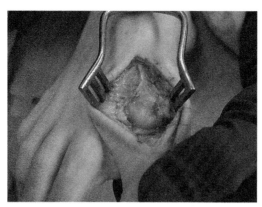

Fig. 4. Passage and suturing of EHB, joint capsule, and extensor hood through the first MTP joint.

with 1 subsequently developing a stress fracture of the second metatarsal, and weakness of the hallux in 8 patients. These investigators concluded that IA is indicated in the treatment of advanced disease and considered a salvage procedure. This recommendation by Lau and Daniels should be taken in context because it was made in comparison to a cheilectomy group that had less statistically significant (P<.001) disease on preoperative radiographs than that in patients who underwent IA. Although these groups of investigators advocated great caution, Hamilton and Hubbard[16] found transfer metatarsalgia in approximately 30% of patients postoperatively to be amenable to orthotic modification for athletic recreation. Still, other international studies have also compared the results of EHB IA and Keller arthroplasty.[19]

In the study by Barca,[20] 12 feet were treated with plantaris tendon interposition through a curved dorsomedial incision with cheilectomy and a 20° to 30° dorsal wedge resection from the proximal phalanx. Using a spherical cutter, a concavity was made in the remaining proximal phalangeal base for placement of the plantaris tendon that postharvest had been rolled into a ball. This configuration was then suture anchored in a cruciate fashion and a mini articulated external fixator applied to maintain joint diastasis during capsular scarring. This study's postoperative period was broken into 3-week segments. The first included the fixator and physical therapy, the second was initiated by fixator removal and passive mobilization, and the third included active mobilization. At an average follow-up period of 21 months, all patients reported good or excellent results and the mean dorsiflexion increased by 44°. Magnetic resonance imaging was performed on 1 patient at 20 and 8 months postoperation on the left and right feet, respectively. The images revealed low signal in T2 and T1 for the presence of connective tissue in the metaplastic phase and a tendon packet rich in granulation tissue and capillaries.[20]

Coughlin and Shurnas[21] reported on the usage of 15- to 20-cm gracilis tendon graft rolled into a sutured 1.5 × 1.5-cm ball as a biologic spacer in 7 patients. This autograft was implanted into a reamed proximal phalanx with a base width of 14 to 16 mm. At an average follow-up period of 42 months, all the patients rated their result as good or excellent, with a mean increase in AOFAS scores from 46 preoperation to 86 postoperation, and the mean dorsiflexion range of motion improved from 9° to 34°. At the tendon harvest site, 1 patient developed a sensory neuroma that was associated with loss of lateral superior calf sensation. It was concluded that the gracilis IA gave excellent pain relief and reliable function of the hallux.

In general, these procedures followed the postoperative protocol: the patient was allowed to weight bear as tolerated in a postoperative rigid-soled shoe for 3 to 4 weeks and was then switched to fully plantigrade weight bearing. Depending on the investigators, early range of motion was encouraged between 10 days and 3 weeks as long as pain and swelling were tolerable.[16–21]

Autograft: Capsular IA

In a retrospective case series, Hahn and colleagues[22] presented 22 patients with grade IV HR who underwent minimal proximal phalanx resection with preservation of the flexor hallucis brevis insertion and medial capsular IA. The joint capsule was elevated off the medial eminence while preserving its distal attachment to the proximal phalanx to create a tongue-shaped flap that was transversely interposed into the joint and sutured to the lateral capsule with an absorbable suture. The joint was then pinned with a 0.062-mm K-wire in 5° of valgus and 10° to 15° of extension for a 3-week duration. A postoperative mean AOFAS hallux MTP-IP score of 77.8 demonstrated clinical improvement and was compared with that of historical control patients who underwent tendinous IA. Alignment and stability were well maintained, and improvement in joint motion was sustained during the 24-month follow-up period. Two patients sustained stress fractures of a lesser metatarsal postoperation, but it was reported that the findings are comparable to those in control patients who underwent tendinous IA.

Autograft: Capsule-Periosteum IA

The rationale for a capsule-periosteum IA in the treatment of HR was presented by Roukis and colleagues[23] as follows:

> Joint capsules and their supporting ligaments are richly supplied by free nerve endings and are the major source of joint sensation, with those regions most subject to compression being particularly heavily innervated. This procedure effectively denervates the first (MTP) by stripping the capsule and periosteum of their innervation while respecting the vascular supply to the first metatarsal, proximal phalanx and sesamoid bones. Thus, this procedure has a distinct advantage over others... (and) renders the first (MTP) insensate.

In addition, these investigators argue that the significant hypertrophy within the capsule and periosteum in HR renders these native tissues ideally positioned and suited for interposition while affording tissue viability and vascular ingrowth. The ideal flap position determined in the study interposed between the plantar surface of the first metatarsal head, and the sesamoid apparatus lends for no development of osseous contact–induced pain.

Roukis and colleagues[23] presented short-term results with a mean follow-up period of 16.8 months for 15 feet with severe HR, which were treated with a distally based flap that was firmly adhered to the undersurface of the metatarsal head through the use of drill holes parallel to the first metatarsal–sesamoid articulation and Kessler-Kleinert locking suture. Patients were preoperatively and postoperatively subjectively evaluated with a modified version of the AOFAS's 100-point Hallux MTP-IP Joint Scale. The study population exhibited subjective patient improvement and satisfaction, increased first MTP joint dorsal range of motion, sustained hallux plantar range of motion and power, and improved radiographic joint space while none developed concomitant deformity or required surgical intervention in the short postoperative period.

Allograft Interposition

Because of donor-site complications and increased length of surgical time, multiple foot and ankle surgeons in the treatment of HR have described the use of allograft IA. Givissis and colleagues[24] published a hallux MTP IA technique using fascia lata allograft for the treatment of HR in the elderly patients or patients with low demand. The joint was inspected dorsally to determine if the procedure would address the visualized pathologic condition. Next, a thin resection ideally not exceeding 10% of the length of the phalanx was performed. A fascia lata allograft was prepared according to the package insert for 5 minutes. Then a 3 × 4-cm piece is cut and folded to form a quadriparallel pack with the corners stitched with 3-0 polyglactin 910 (Vicryl). The cut spacer is then placed, the surrounding soft tissues are balanced, the graft is removed temporarily to introduce a 1.6-mm K-wire, the allograft is placed, and a K-wire is driven in a retrograde fashion through the spacer to the metatarsal shaft level. Postclosure, patients were able to heel weight bear on the first postoperative day. The K-wire is removed 6 weeks postoperation.

Overall, it was related that the procedure is not technically demanding, is easily reproducible, allows for immediate weight bearing, and is suitable for the elderly and smokers who carry an increased risk of arthrodesis failure. A single-center prospective study has been initiated to validate the long-term clinical outcomes of this method. In the study by Givissis and colleagues,[24] the 1-year follow-up results in 11 cases were good to excellent, according to both the AOFAS scores and the patients' satisfaction. There was no further elaboration regarding objective measures or complications.

Not all researchers, however, agree on the benefits of fascia lata graft because of some its concerning drawbacks, including limited supply, lack of pliability, and susceptibility to tearing.[4] The first reported use of acellular dermis processed from human cadaveric skin as a spacer at the first MTP joint was, in brief as a technique tip, by Kolker and Weinfeld in 2007.[25] In their technique, they used a 2 × 7-cm piece of AlloDerm (LifeCell Corporation, Branchburg, NJ, USA) rolled into a 2 × 2-cm ball that was sutured onto itself and then placed in situ after resection of metatarsal osteophytes and the proximal phalanx. The AlloDerm "anchovy" is then sutured to the inner side of the joint capsule as a K-wire is advanced across the arthroplasty site into the first metatarsal shaft. This step is followed by a standard closure and application of a postoperative shoe, although the patient remained non–weight-bearing for the first 3 days. Thereafter, patients may continue with protected weight bearing for 4 weeks until the K-wire is removed and range of motion exercises are started. The study[25] does not provide information on follow-up and surgical numbers regarding the amount of patients treated with this protocol.

Berlet and colleagues[26] described in detail a surgical technique for IA (**Figs. 5** and **6**) using GRAFTJACKET (Wright Medical Technology, Inc, Arlington, TN, USA), a human acellular dermal regenerative tissue matrix (RTM), as a spacer to mitigate drawbacks from previous techniques. GRAFTJACKET is processed in a way that destroys all immunologic components, minimizes the destruction of the original human dermis, and preserves the vascular channels of the cadaveric dermis and the extracellular matrix contents of elastin, proteoglycans, laminin, tenascin, and collagen types I, III, IV, and VIII. These properties allow rapid revascularization and cellular repopulation and maintenance of tensile strength, and thus, GRAFTJACKET was deemed a good candidate for joint surfacing.[4] In a retrospective review of 9 consecutive patients with Coughlin grade III HR, Berlet and colleagues reported on the outcomes of RTM IA with an average follow-up period of 12.7 months. They followed a stepwise

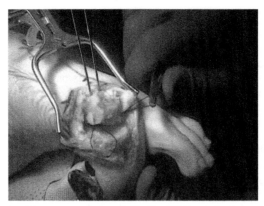

Fig. 5. Distal metatarsal bone tunnels are drilled and 2 Hewson suture passers are used to accept the graft suture.

procedure that included cheilectomy, metatarsal-sesamoid joint mobilization, modified Keller osteotomy, contouring of the metatarsal head, RTM preparation, IA, and closure. Careful attention must be directed at placing the reticular layer, or "shiny side," against the metatarsal head to orient the vascular supply to the appropriate tissue as well as when creating 2 bone tunnels for tight apposition and fixation with 0-Vicryl. After the operation, patients were allowed to heel weight bear as tolerated. There were no reported complications or failures, and the mean total AOFAS score significantly increased from an average of 63.9 preoperation to 87.9 postoperation. Berlet and colleagues[26] postulated that the excellent early results and lack of complications might be because of the minimization of bone resection, the lack of donor-site comorbidities, the resurfacing of the sesamoid articulation, and the maintenance of the intrinsics. In summary, the investigators stated on this technique as "may offer the young and active patient with advanced HR an opportunity to maintain an active lifestyle, while retaining the possibility for more surgical options should the condition progress."

In a recent poster abstract presented at American College of Foot and Ankle Surgeons and AOFAS, 6 of these original 9 patients were available for follow-up.

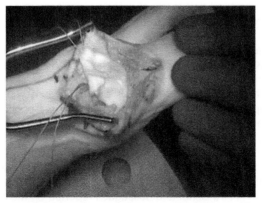

Fig. 6. The remaining graft is brought around to cover the metatarsal head. The graft is tied into the existing dorsal sutures. Excess graft is then trimmed.

The outcome measures for the group were tracked retrospectively with an average follow-up period of 5.43 years. These measures included AOFAS scores modified for pain and function with a maximum of 68 points, reoperation rates, and overall satisfaction with the procedure. Hyer and colleagues[27] found that no patient had a subsequent fusion or required an additional procedure on the first MTP joint. Average modified AOFAS scores were 38 (34–43) preoperation versus 65.8 (58–68) postoperation. All patients were satisfied with their results. Similar to the initial study and given the results, it was regarded that RTM IA is a viable alternative to arthrodesis in the active patient with advanced HR.

Brigido and colleagues[4] published the results of 2 case studies in which GRAFT-JACKET was used in 1 patient on the talar dome and in another at the first metatarsal head for joint resurfacing, with a 2-year follow-up period. Their article begins with a historical perspective on cutis allograft and xenograft arthroplasty, with a mention of previously used membranes for joints including chromicized pig bladder, cellophane, and nylon. However, with the advent of biologic allograft scaffolds, the use of cutis has dissipated. In this study, 52-year-old female patient with HR underwent IA after using a cup-and-cone reaming system, with a conical preparation of the metatarsal head and cup preparation of the proximal phalanx base for acceptance of hemiarthroplasty. Next, 2 vertical trephine holes were drilled for the bioscaffold attachment after it was wrapped around the head in a hoodlike fashion and secured around the metatarsal neck in an under-and-over technique. Finally, a hemi-implant was placed in the base of the proximal phalanx.

Brigido and colleagues[4] had made no mention of the postoperative protocol for this patient; however, it is noted that the patient had less pain and more function until the 18th month when the patient presented with tenderness of the first interspace. An open biopsy was performed, and on joint exposure, there was visualization of an articular surface with smooth, shiny, hyalinelike appearance. Histologic analysis of the metatarsal head revealed a significant layer of mature neocartilage adjacent to the subchondral bone with differentiated chondrocytes throughout the matrix of the acellular human dermal bioscaffold. Thus, the findings confirm that RTM bioscaffold is able to accept host chondrocytes. In addition, a joint surface can be formed that acts and functions in a way similar to that of native articular cartilage. Although this finding is profound, the investigators did not address how they treated the patient's tenderness intraoperatively or after the second procedure and if it resolved or not.

Although long-term randomized controlled trials are lacking for IA, the reported short- and mid-term results are at least comparable and more often exceed the alternatives for treatment of end-stage HR. This treatment option for young patients with HR may exceedingly become commonplace in the future.

ARTHRODIASTASIS

The word arthrodiastasis is derived from the Greek *arthro* meaning joint, *dia* meaning through, and *tasis* meaning to stretch out. In terms of orthopedic procedures, it was first used in Verona, Italy, in 1979 to describe articulated hip distraction; however, more than a century earlier, the term was used to describe similar techniques. The primary focus of this group of procedures is to restore function to a stiff ankylosed joint through a staged lengthening of shortened ligaments and fibrotic capsule. In the process, the functional range of motion of the joint increases gradually, both intrinsic and extrinsic muscular imbalances are reduced, and the distraction of the articular surfaces helps to protect the cartilage from further destruction.[28,29] In addition, microangiogenesis in the soft tissue around the joint that is undergoing diastasis assists in the reparative process with enhancement of the synovial nutrition and state of hyperviscosity.[29]

Early Results

Thomas[28] published on the use of distraction to ensure postoperative distraction of the hallux after the Keller arthroplasty for the treatment of HR and valgus. The study asserted "traction in one form or another is usually applied to the part of the limb distal to the arthroplasty, with the object of maintaining an adequate gap at the false joint during the first few weeks of healing" and Thomas, along with other surgeons of the time, thought this to be a desirable addition to arthroplasties used for the treatment of HR. Although pulp traction, via a pin or nylon suture, was most commonly performed, it was recommended to keep the MTP joint distracted to a greater degree to prevent spontaneous regression through the use of an intramedullary wire or external staple. After completion of Keller arthroplasty in a standard format, a 0.062-in K-wire with a trocar point is inserted while the toe is pulled distally to maintain the maximum gap at the arthroplasty site. The wire is cut one-eighth of an inch beyond the distal tip of the hallux and, with the aid of a Gelpi or Jackson Burrows retractor to hold the toe to length, the skin is closed. After retractor removal, tincture of benzoin is placed, and while this is wet, a sterile wood-wool bandage is applied. The other option was diastasis by using an external staple. After arthroplasty, 2 small medial stab incisions were made; 1 at the level of the metatarsal neck and the other at the neck of the proximal phalanx. A sharp awl, or drill, is then passed through the stab incisions to make transverse holes for placement of a K-wire that is bent into the shape of a staple. A similar dressing is applied as previously described. After both of these operations, patients were retained in hospital, on average, 4 to 5 days and instructed to remain non–weight-bearing until the 10th day at which time, patients can walk on their plasters. Three weeks after surgery, the casts were removed, sutures excised, and the wires removed with pliers.[28]

In total, Thomas reviewed 271 operations with the following complications: 7 patients with delayed wound healing, 1 with infection, 1 with persistent swelling, 1 with pulmonary embolus, 4 with pin-tract sepsis, 1 with OA of the IP joint, 2 with "Mastisol" dermatitis (before changing protocol), 8 contractures of the extensor hallucis longus, 1 bony fusion of the MTP joint, and 1 avascular necrosis of the proximal phalanx. The results were evaluated as excellent in 40%, good in 47%, and poor in 13%, while patients were pleased or satisfied 96% of the time with only 4% being dissatisfied. In the long-term review of 139 patients who had undergone operation on 193 feet with a minimum follow-up period of 12 months, it was concluded that the long-term results of "modified arthroplasties... appeared to be better than the results of the standard operation," with the external staple producing better gap maintenance and the intermedullary placement of the K-wire producing better overall end results.[28]

In a prospective trial by Sherman and colleagues,[30] 35 patients underwent 51 Keller arthroplasty procedures; yet, only 8 procedures were for the indication of HR. In this comparison, group A underwent standard Keller arthroplasty followed by gathering of the synovium into the space with a polyglycolic acid (Dexon) purse-string suture. Correction was held with a wool and crepe bandage. Group B had the same procedure with the exception of the synovial purse-string suture; the group did receive an intermedullary K-wire that was driven to the metatarsal head. Both groups had wound checks at 2.5 weeks after operation, with discontinuation of the sutures and K-wire removal. The power of flexion of the hallux after operation was statistically different between the groups, with reduction by an average of 30% in the wired group. In addition, the wired group exhibited more radiographic evidence of degeneration postoperatively, without increase in the size of the arthroplasty gap. It was summarized that patients disliked the wire, and there was neither reduction in postoperative pain nor improvement in healing or quality of the anatomic result.

Recent Results

Within the past 5 years, additional research has emerged that, in comparison to older research, shows better clinical and functional results. Talarico and colleagues[29] studied the effectiveness of arthrodiastasis at the hallux MTP joint for the treatment of HR in 133 patients over a 6-year period. Using the AOFAS hallux MTP-IJ scale and radiologic findings, patients were evaluated at 3, 6, 9, and 12 months postoperation. Their surgical protocol consisted of cheilectomy of the metatarsal head with the application of a straight monolateral fixator. Acute distraction consisted of up to 5 mm and was confirmed with fluoroscopy. The joint was then left static for 5 to 7 days, after which, the patients performed distraction of 0.5 mm per day for 14 days to account for 8 and 12 mm of total distraction. The joint was then left static for 14 more days before removal of the fixator, after which, physical therapy for range of motion exercises was initiated.

The results of this arthrodiastasis at the hallux MTP joint included an average 3-month AOFAS score of 83 that steadily increased to 88 at 12 months. Early postoperative total range of motion in 119 of 133 patients (89%) was more than twice their preoperative value. In addition, the first MTP joint space increased in 115 patients (86%) from 1.8 mm preoperatively to 5.2 mm postoperatively. Only 1 patient required arthrodesis in the initial 12-month follow-up, whereas none of the 9 patients with implants and a fixator that was applied without opening the joint preoperatively required removal of the implant. The average AOFAS score at 3-year follow-up was 78 for 44 of the 133 patients. In this long-term follow-up group, 3 patients underwent arthrodesis and 1 received a 2-piece first MTP joint implant, which were all performed at other facilities.

Reize and colleagues[31] investigated whether K-wire transfixation or distraction following Keller-Brandes arthroplasty fared better postoperatively in the treatment of HR. The treatment protocol was conducted on 71 feet with HR in patients older than 50 years and who had marked degenerative changes. The surgical approach was via a straight midline medial incision, followed by the preparation of a proximally based medial capsule flap, removal of the proximal phalanx at the metaphyseal-diaphyseal junction (approximately one-third of its length), and evaluation of the alignment and cerclage fibreux. Next, K-wire transfixation was performed to the level of the midmetatarsal or distraction was performed with another wire in the distal phalanx of the hallux. The wound was then closed. Patients received plaster casting in the distraction group, and only firm-soled shoes in the transfixation group; all wires remained in place for 21 days, after which, all the patients received firm-soled shoes for the next 3 weeks and night splints for the first 3 months following operation. Of the original 71 patients treated, only 14 of the 33 patients in the distraction group and 12 of the 38 patients in the transfixation group presented for follow-up clinical and radiographic examination. Although the patient number is less, the mean combined (patients with procedure indicated for HR as well as hallux valgus) subset follow-up time was 9.1 years. In a follow-up questionnaire, only 83.3% of patients treated with K-wire transfixation related no pain, whereas this number was 92.9% in the distraction group. Those who reported pain related that it was mild. Mean hallux dorsiflexion and plantar flexion were 1° and 6° greater in the distraction group, respectively. No unstable joints were encountered in the K-wire group, but there was one completely stiff hallux. Meanwhile, there was instability in 14% of patients treated with distraction. Overall, patient satisfaction was high with a very good or good result in 88% of the distraction group and 83% of the transfixation group. However, when directly questioned about cosmetic results, dissatisfaction increased to 18.7% in the distraction and 33% in the transfixation groups.

In the study by Reize and colleagues,[31] arthrodiastasis resulted in better outcomes in satisfaction with less adjacent joint destruction but had higher rates of instability than transfixation. These findings are consistent with those in the study by Talarico and colleagues[29] when they conclude, "distraction across the joint allows for the relief of abnormal pressures, forces, and muscular imbalances that cause destructive jamming of the first metatarsophalangeal joint." Simultaneously, diastasis creates an environment that promotes angiogenesis and reparative processes.

DISCUSSION

Unfortunately, regarding HR, the only real consensus in the literature is that no conservative treatment can reverse the progressive disease process but a course of this treatment needs to be undertaken before surgical intervention. In most circles, arthrodesis is still the gold standard. This apart, there is no consensus about the treatment of painful advanced degenerative arthrosis involving the first MTP joint. Therefore, the authors think that it is critically important to stratify patients based on diagnosis, age, and activity level and carry on a frank discussion with patients to best identify their goals and desires before operative intervention. They also consider that one must focus on treating the symptoms rather than the radiographs. Young to middle-aged, active patients with HR should be considered candidates for the procedures described earlier because they all minimize bony resection, provide symptomatic relief, and maintain or restore motion and strength. Most notably in this population, these procedures do not seem to replace those procedures that are well documented in traditional resectional arthroplasty, arthrodesis, and joint replacement. If any of the procedures presented in this article fail, the procedure can then be revised, most often, to an arthrodesis without concern over length, the need for graft, and the concern over fusing an additional osseous interface.

Comparing Results

Mann and Oates[32] believed "the critical elements in an analysis of results should be the long-term relief of pain, improvement in joint motion and the avoidance of complications." The authors concur with this statement. To the authors' knowledge and given the outcomes reporting on the procedures discussed earlier, the AOFAS hallux MTP-IP joint score is the most appropriate subjective yet numerical value to report outcomes. This score was most commonly used to describe a study's postoperative state and at times, was included in a preoperative description of the study populations. This 100-point scale is composed of separate sections for pain (40 points), function (45 points), and alignment (15 points) (**Table 1**).[33] Given the scoring scale, after arthrodesis, the highest attainable AOFAS score is 90. A comparison of the studies referenced within this article that used the AOFAS MTP-IP joint scoring system is compiled and presented in **Table 2**.

Considerations

To aid the foot and ankle surgeon in clinical and surgical decision making, as well as compare results from the literature, classifications have been created. Although the Coughlin classification is the most utilized at present, many different classifications, including Hattrup and Johnson classification and author-specific modifications, were used throughout the studies discussed herein that make direct comparison of indications both frustrating and impossible. Doing so could only be done if a great deal of information was implied.

Table 1
The AOFAS's Hallux MTP-IP Joint Scale

Characteristic	Description	Assigned Value (Points)
Pain	No pain	40
40 Possible	Mild, occasional	30
	Moderate, daily	20
	Severe, almost always present	0
Function	Activity limitations	
45 Possible	No limitation	10
	Limitation of recreation but not daily or job-related activities	7
		4
	Limitation of daily activities and recreation	0
	Severe limitation of daily activities and recreation	
	Footwear requirements	
	Fashionable and conventional shoes with no insert required	10
		5
	Ability to wear only comfortable shoes or the need for an insert	0
	Need to wear modified shoes or a brace	
	First MTP joint motion: dorsiflexion plus plantar flexion	
	≥75°	10
	30°–74°	5
	<30°	0
	First IP joint motion: plantar flexion	
	No restriction	5
	<10°	0
	MTP-IP joint stability: in all directions	
	Stable	5
	Definitely unstable or able to dislocate	0
	Callus related to MTP & IP joint stability	
	Absent or asymptomatic callus	5
	Symptomatic callus	0
Alignment	Good, hallux well aligned	15
15 Possible	Fair, some hallux malalignment observed but no symptoms	8
		0
	Poor, obvious symptomatic malalignment	
100 Points possible		

Data from Kitaoka H, Alexander I, Adelaar R, et al. Clinical rating systems for the ankle-hindfoot, midfoot, hallux, and lesser toes. Foot Ankle Int 1994;15:349.

As previously stated, the authors appreciate the credence of a patient's subjective complaints, desires, and goals over an arbitrary classification system when choosing surgical intervention if it is determined necessary. The authors, however, do realize the importance of knowing and practicing the standard of care; therefore, they have classified patients with HR based on the Coughlin classification: grade I has less than 50% loss of motion with only a dorsal osteophyte on radiographic examination, grade II has moderate radiographic joint narrowing, grade III has 75% to 100% loss of MTP joint range of motion and substantial joint space narrowing on radiographic examination, and grade IV has the characteristics of grade III plus pain at the mid–range of motion.[3]

Table 2
Comparison of AOFAS scores from studies discussed herein

	Coughlin and Shurnas[3] Comparison	Lau and Daniels[18] Comparison	Schenk and Colleagues[19] Comparison	Tendinous IA	Capsular IA	Acellular Matrix IA	Arthrodiastasis
	Cheilectomy (N = 110)	Cheilectomy (N = 24)	Keller arthroplasty (N = 30)	Hamilton and Hubbard[16] EHB IA (N = 37)	Hahn and colleagues[22] (N = 22)	Berlet and colleagues[26] (N = 9)	Talarico and colleagues[29] at 12 mo (N = 133)
Preoperation	45 (24–70)	NA	50	64.2	NA	64 (44–72)	NA
Postoperation	90 (67–100)	78 (65–91)	88	95.4	77.8	88 (72–100)	88
	Arthrodesis (N = 30)	EHB IA (N = 11)	EHB IA (N = 22)	Coughlin and Shurnas[21] gracilis IA (N = 7)	—	Hyer and colleagues[33] at 5.43 y (N = 6)	Talarico and colleagues[29] at 3 y (N = 44)
Preoperation	38 (24–60)	NA	57	46	—	38 (34–43)[a]	NA
Postoperation	89 (72–90)	72 (56–88)	89	86	—	66 (58–68)[a]	78

All values are given as the mean, with the range in parentheses.
Abbreviations: N, number of feet; NA, not available.
[a] An AOFAS score on a modified scale selective for pain and function, with a maximum total score of 68 points.

Generally the authors favor cheilectomy for symptomatic grade I and grade II HR because it is a joint-preserving procedure, improves MTP joint range of motion, and reduces pain with little long-term consequences and without limiting traditional procedures. For these same reasons, the authors embrace resurfacing, IA, and arthrodiastasis of the hallux MTP joint in the treatment of patients with grade III HR with less than 50% of the articular surface of the first metatarsal head at the time of intervention. Whereas, in grade III HR with more than 50% of cartilage destruction and grade IV HR the authors concur with the findings of the studies by Coughlin and Shurnas[3] that these patients should be treated with arthrodesis.

For those patients with more than 50% of their metatarsal head cartilage remaining, joint resurfacing and diastasis techniques are viable treatment options in the foot and ankle surgeon's armamentarium. Theoretically, these procedures forego the need for removal of painful hardware, reduce the incidence of recurrence because they are addressing the pathologic condition, and add a barrier or mechanism to prevent chondrolysis. Because long-term absolute stability is not needed in any of these procedures, cases of delayed union and nonunion should be less painful.

Standardization in evaluation and grading is needed to adequately evaluate preoperatively, to make an informed operative decision based on evidence-based medicine outcomes, and to effectively compare postoperative results on a short-, medium-, and long-term basis. Until then and higher levels of evidence-based medicine results are available, it is not possible to endorse any of the discussed procedures over another. Each procedure has its place, and the authors appreciate of having the procedures as viable easy-to-implement options for surgical patients with HR.

REFERENCES

1. Hamilton WG, O'Malley MJ, Thompson FM, et al. Capsular interposition arthroplasty for severe hallux rigidus. Foot Ankle Int 1997;18(2):68–70.
2. Easley ME, Davis WH, Anderson RB. Intermediate to long-term follow-up of medial-approach dorsal cheilectomy for hallux rigidus. Foot Ankle Int 1999;20:147–52.
3. Coughlin MJ, Shurnas PS. Hallux rigidus: grading & long-term results of operative treatment. J Bone Joint Surg Am 2003;85(11):2072–88.
4. Brigido SA, Troiano M, Schoenhaus H. Biologic resurfacing of the ankle and first metatarsophalangeal joint: case studies with a 2-year follow-up. Clin Podiatr Med Surg 2009;26:633–45.
5. Title CI, Zaret D, Means KR, et al. First metatarsal head OATS technique: an approach to cartilage damage. Foot Ankle Int 2006;27(11):1000–2.
6. Davies MS, Saxby TS. Arthroscopy of the first metatarsophalangeal joint. J Bone Joint Surg Br 1999;81:203–6.
7. Debnath UK, Hemmady MV, Hariharan K. Indications for and technique of first metatarsal joint arthroscopy. Foot Ankle Int 2006;27(12):1049–54.
8. Ritsila V, Santavirta S, Alhopuro, et al. Periosteal and perichondral grafting in reconstructive surgery. Clin Orthop Relat Res 1994;302:259–65.
9. Jamora H, Ritsila V. Reconstruction of patellar cartilage defects with free periosteal grafts. Scand J Plast Reconstr Surg 1987;21:175.
10. Ritsila V, Eskola A, Hoikka V, et al. Periosteal resurfacing of the metatarsal head in hallux rigidus and Freiberg's disease. J Orthop Rheum 1992;5:79–84.
11. Hopson M, Stone P, Paden M. First metatarsal head osteoarticular transfer system for salvage of a failed hemicap-implant: a case report. J Foot Ankle Surg 2009;48(4):2009.

12. Kravitz AB. Osteochondral autogenous transplantation for an osteochondral defect of the first metatarsal head: a case resport. J Foot Ankle Surg 2005; 44(2):152–5.

13. Miyamoto W, Takao M, Uchio Y, et al. Late-state Freiberg disease treated by osteochondral plug transplantation: a case series. Foot Ankle Int 2008;29(9): 950–5.

14. Zelent ME, Neese DJ. Osteochondral autograft transfer of the first metatarsal head: a case report. J Foot Ankle Surg 2005;44(5):406–11.

15. DeHeer PA. The case against first metatarsal phalangeal joint implant arthroplasty. Clin Podiatr Med Surg 2006;23:709–23.

16. Hamilton WG, Hubbard CE. Hallux rigidus: excisional arthroplasty. Foot Ankle Clin 2000;5(3):663–71.

17. Kennedy JG, Brodsky AR, Gradl G, et al. Outcomes after interposition arthroplasty for treatment of hallux rigidus. Clin Orthop Relat Res 2006;445: 210–5.

18. Lau JT, Daniels TR. Outcomes following cheilectomy and interpositional arthroplasty in hallux rigidus. Foot Ankle Int 2001;22(6):462–70.

19. Schenk S, Meizer R, Kramer R, et al. Resection arthroplasty with and without capsular interposition for treatment of severe hallux rigidus. Int Orthop 2009;33: 145–50.

20. Barca F. Tendon arthroplasty of the first metatarsophalangeal joint in hallux rigidus: preliminary communication. Foot Ankle Int 1997;18(4):222–8.

21. Coughlin MJ, Shurnas PJ. Soft-tissue arthroplasty for hallux rigidus. Foot Ankle Int 2003;24(9):661–72.

22. Hahn MP, Gerhardt N, Thordarson DB. Medial capsular interpositional arthroplasty for severe hallux rigidus. Foot Ankle Int 2009;30(6):494–9.

23. Roukis TS, Landsman AS, Ringstrom, et al. Distally based capsule-periosteum interpositional arthroplasty for hallux rigidus: indications, operative technique and short-term follow-up. J Am Podiatr Med Assoc 2003;93(5):349–66.

24. Givissis P, Symeonidis P, Christodoulou A, et al. Interposition arthroplasty of the first metatarsophalangeal joint with a fascia lata allograft. J Am Podiatr Med Assoc 2008;98(2):160–3.

25. Kolker D, Weinfeld S. Technique tip: a modification to the keller arthroplasty using interposition allograft. Foot Ankle Int 2007;28(2):266–8.

26. Berlet GC, Hyer CF, Lee TH, et al. Interpositional arthroplasty of the first MTP joint using a regenerative tissue matrix for the treatment of advanced hallux rigidus. Foot Ankle Int 2008;29(1):10–21.

27. Hyer CF, Granata JD, Berlet GC, et al. Interpositional arthroplasty of the first metatarsophalangeal joint using a regenerative tissue matrix for the treatment of advanced hallux rigidus: 5 year case series follow-up. Podium presentation at the American Orthopaedic Foot & Ankle Society (AOFAS) 26th National Meeting. National Harbor (MD), July 7–10, 2010. Poster presentation at the American College of Foot and Ankle Surgeons (ACFAS) 68th Annual Scientific Conference. Las Vegas (NV), February 22–26, 2010.

28. Thomas FB. Keller's arthroplasty modified: a technique to ensure post-operative distraction of the toe. J Bone Joint Surg Br 1962;44(2):356–65.

29. Talarico LM, Vito GR, Goldstein L, et al. Management of hallux limitus with distraction of the first metatarsophalangeal joint. J Am Podiatr Med Assoc 2005;95(2): 121–9.

30. Sherman KP, Douglas DL, Benson MK. Keller's arthroplasty: is distraction useful? A prospective trial. J Bone Joint Surg Br 1984;66(5):765–9.

31. Reize P, Schanbacher J, Wulker N. K-wire transfixation or distraction following the Keller-Brandes arthroplasty in Hallux rigidus and Hallux valgus? Int Orthop 2007; 31:325–31.

32. Mann RA, Oates JC. Arthrodesis of the first metatarsophalangeal joint. Foot Ankle 1980;1:159–66.

33. Kitaoka H, Alexander I, Adelaar R, et al. Clinical rating systems for the ankle-hindfoot, midfoot, hallux, and lesser toes. Foot Ankle Int 1994;15:349.

Current Concepts and Techniques in Foot and Ankle Surgery

First Metatarsophalangeal Joint Arthrodesis: Current Fixation Options

Jared L. Moon, DPM[a],*, Michael C. McGlamry, DPM[a,b]

KEYWORDS

- First metatarsophalangeal joint arthrodesis • Hallux rigidus
- Hallux limitus • Fixation

Broca was first to describe the first metatarsophalangeal joint (MTPJ) arthrodesis procedure in 1852.[1] In 1894, Clutton[2] showed good results with the procedure, but little was published after his paper until 1941 when McKeever[3] revived interest in the procedure. Since McKeever,[3] there have been many publications on the procedure, all showing high fusion rates with various types of fixation used.[4–15]

One possible complication of first MTPJ arthrodesis is nonunion.[16] During gait, up to 90% of the body's weight is transferred through the first MTPJ,[17] which makes rigid fixation of the arthrodesis site a necessity. As with any fusion procedure, the goal of fixation is the same: maintain the position of the arthrodesis site until osseous consolidation occurs. As Perren[18] stated, it is a race between bone healing and fixation failure. Given the numerous fixation options available for first MTPJ arthrodesis, it is worth taking an evidence-based approach and reviewing the literature to see what fixation options are recommended for this procedure.

CURRENT FIXATION OPTIONS
Kirschner Wire/Steinman Pin Fixation

Perhaps the most frequently reported and simplest of fixation techniques for first MTPJ arthrodesis is with the use of Kirschner wires (K-wires) or Steinmann pins.[19–22] Regardless of technological advances in fixation, the literature shows that K-wire or Steinman pin fixation is an acceptable fixation option. Mann and Oates[4] published a study in 1980 on 41 feet with a 95% fusion rate using 2 threaded Steinmann pins. In 1984, Mann and Thompson[22] used the Steinmann pin fixation technique with a 94% fusion rate on 18 feet.

Disclosure: Michael McGlamry, DPM, serves as a consultant surgeon on the advisory board for Orthohelix and BME.
a DeKalb Medical Center, Decatur, GA, USA
b Podiatry Institute, Decatur, GA, USA
* Corresponding author.
E-mail address: jared.l.moon@gmail.com

Niskanen and colleagues[5] in 1993 showed successful fusion in 34/39 joints with the use of both biodegradable rods and K-wires. There were 3 clinical nonunions using biodegradable rods and 5 radiographic nonunions. The K-wire group had no clinical nonunions and 3 radiographic nonunions. Smith and colleagues[23] used multiple threaded 0.062 K-wires to successfully fuse 97% of 34 feet. Again, high fusion rates are found using both K-wire and Steinmann pin fixation.

Biomechanical studies comparing K-wire and Steinmann pin fixation with more advanced forms of fixation, such as plates and screws, are rare. In a cadaveric study in 1993, Curtis and colleagues[24] assessed both strength and rigidity, comparing 3 different fixation techniques: crossed K-wires, a single interfragmentary screw, and a dorsal plate. Of these constructs, interfragmentary screw fixation was found to be the most stable when subjected to cyclic loading.

A similar cadaveric study by Rongstad and colleagues[25] compared 4 different fixation techniques, including 4.0-mm oblique Arbeitsgemeinschaft fur Osteosynthesefragen (AO) cancellous screw, a miniplate dorsally, oblique 4.5-mm Herbert cannulated screw, and a 3/32 Steinmann pin placed longitudinally. Except for the 4.0-mm AO screw construct, each fixation method was supplement with an oblique 0.045 K-wire. Each specimen was tested to failure. Both the plate and Herbert screw were found to be stronger constructs than the AO screw or Steinmann pin. The Steinmann pin was found have no significant difference in strength compared with the AO screw.

Politi and colleagues[16] in 2003 compared the biomechanical stability 4 different fixation techniques, including an interfragmentary compression screw, crossed 0.062 K-wires, a 4-hole dorsal miniplate, and a 4-hole dorsal miniplate with an interfragmentary compression screw. Their results showed that the dorsal miniplate without an interfragmentary compression screw and crossed K-wires were the weakest constructs, whereas the plate with an interfragmentary screw was the most stable construct.

Although high fusion rates have been observed with both K-wire and Steinmann pin fixation, there are still questions surrounding their biomechanical strength compared with that of other available methods of fixation. The study by Rongstad and colleagues[25] did show similar strength of a longitudinally placed Steinmann pin compared with AO screw fixation. One possibility is that the increased diameter of the Steinmann pin gives it an advantage compared with that of a K-wire, or the increased strength of this construct could be caused by its longitudinal position. If the preferred method of fixating the first MTPJ is to use crossed K-wires, it may be worth considering adding a K-wire in a longitudinal position, as shown in **Fig. 1**. One potential issue when using a longitudinal pin or wire is that interphalangeal joint arthritis may result.[26]

Screw Fixation

Screw fixation is a commonly used method for fixating the first MTPJ when adequate bone stock is available. Various fixation constructs have been described all leading to acceptable fusion rates. Wassink and Martin[6] in 2009 fused 109 joints, with a 95% fusion rate. They used a single-screw construct with an AO 3.5-mm partially threaded screw inserted in oblique fashion from the metatarsal proximally/medially into the proximal phalanx distally/laterally. Seventy-eight percent of the feet required removal of the screw after surgery.[6] Placing the head of the screw in the metaphyseal flare of the metatarsal helps prevent the need for further removal of the screw.[27]

Brodsky and colleagues[7] in 2005 had a 100% fusion rate using screws on 60 feet. Two 3.5-mm cortical screws were used. Both were inserted in parallel fashion from the proximal dorsal aspect of the metatarsal to the plantar distal aspect of the proximal phalanx. Hyer and colleagues[8] in 2008 had a 92.9% fusion rate using 4.0-mm partially threaded screws in standard crossing fashion.

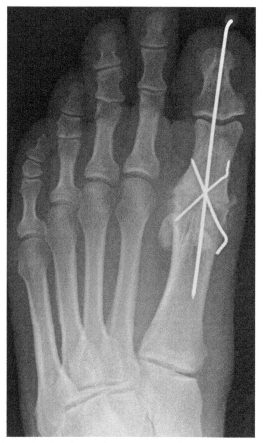

Fig. 1. Crossed 0.062 K-wire fixation with 0.062 K-wire longitudinally. (*Courtesy of* Thomas A. Brosky, DPM, GA.)

Few biomechanical studies comparing different screw orientations to fuse the first MTPJ exist. In one such study Molloy and colleagues[28] compared 2 crossed, 4.0-mm, partially threaded cannulated cancellous screws with an intramedullary technique described by Hansen[29] using a 6.5-mm partially threaded cancellous screw. Their results showed that the intramedullary technique provided a significantly stiffer construct compared with the crossed-screw technique. The intramedullary technique was 50% stronger than the crossed-screw technique, although not statistically significant.[28] Although the intramedullary technique may be less commonly used by surgeons to fixate the first MTPJ, the screw's orientation being perpendicular to the arthrodesis site explains its inherent biomechanical strength.[28] A similar increase in biomechanical strength was found when using an intramedullary Steinmann pin in the study by Rongstad and colleagues,[25] as mentioned earlier.

The study by Rongstad and colleagues[25] investigated another biomechanical relationship. They compared a 4.0-mm oblique AO cancellous screw construct with that of an obliquely placed 4.5-mm Herbert cannulated screw supplemented with an oblique 0.045 K-wire. The Herbert screw construct was found to be significantly stronger in force to failure compared with that of the AO screw.[25] This finding is unexpected because the hollow-core design of the cannulated screw tends to lower the pull-out strength of the screw compared with a noncannulated screw with a nonhollow core.[30] The biomechanical strength of a Herbert screw has been compared with that of a 4.0-mm cancellous AO screw in the setting of cadaveric scaphoid bones. Results of this study showed a significant larger compressive load generated by the 4.0-mm cancellous AO screw compared with that of the Herbert screw.[31]

First MTPJ arthrodesis with screw fixation leads to acceptable fusion rates. One biomechanical study shows that placing screws parallel to the fusion site leads to the most stable construct, and another biomechanical study shows that a single crossed Herbert screw was stronger than a 4.0-mm oblique cancellous screw. More biomechanical studies need to be done on screw orientation before conclusions can be drawn on superiority of a given screw construct orientation.

Plate Fixation

Plate fixation of the first MTPJ has traditionally been used by orthopedists. Few studies have been published in which plate fixation alone is used on a patient population. All the studies available to date are of nonlocking plate technology rather than locking plate technology, as shown in **Fig. 2**. Fusion rates for first MTPJ arthrodesis with nonlocking plate fixation seem to be comparable with other forms of fixation.

Bennett and colleagues[9] in 2009 fused 233 joints using a nonlocking 5-hole plate secured with 3.5-mm and 4.0-mm cancellous screws. No interfragmentary compression screws were used. The fusion rate was 98.7% with no plates breaking and only 3

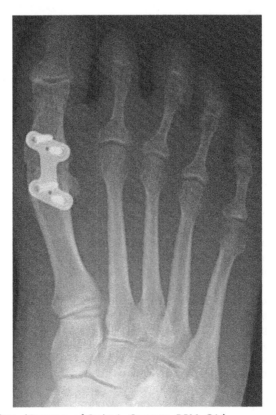

Fig. 2. Locking plate. (*Courtesy of* Craig A. Camasta, DPM, GA.)

patients requiring hardware removal. These investigators had previously reported on the same procedure using a hand set for fixation and had a 13% nonunion rate, leading them to search for a better way to fixate the first MTPJ.[32]

Other investigators have reported success with plating the first MTPJ. Hyer and colleagues[8] in 2008 published a 90.3% fusion rate on 31 joints using a low-profile, 5-hole, nonlocking titanium plate with only 1 patient requiring revision. In this study, the investigators compared the fusion rate of the plate with a crossed-screw construct and found similar fusion rates using both constructs.[8] Coughlin fused 58 joints using a 6-hole, nonlocking, vitallium plating system. No compression screw was used in this study, but occasionally the fusion site was augmented with a K-wire. A 98% fusion rate was achieved with nonunion and breakage occurring in 2% of feet, delayed union in 2%, and plate removal was necessary in 7% of patients.[33]

Biomechanical studies comparing different types of plating systems are lacking, therefore it is difficult to draw conclusions on the strength of the different plating systems available. In addition, no studies are available comparing nonlocking with locking plating constructs for first MTPJ arthrodesis.

Rongstad and colleagues,[25] as previously mentioned, found a miniplate construct with no interfragmentary compression screw to be superior in both force to failure and stiffness compared with that of an AO screw, Herbert screw, and Steinmann pin fixation. The miniplate used was a 6-hole, nonlocking, vitallium plate using 2.7-mm nonlocking screws.[25]

The biomechanical study by Politi and colleagues[16] concerned various fixation constructs, and produced results contradicting the findings of Rongstad and colleagues.[25] Their study showed that fixation of the first MTPJ using only a plate and no compression screw is the weakest construct compared with various techniques including K-wires, screws, and a plate with an interfragmentary compression screw. The plate used was a 4-hole, nonlocking, vitallium plate with 3.5-mm nonlocking screws. The investigators attributed this result to the positioning of the plate. The plate is applied dorsally to the tension side rather than to the plantar surface or compression side.[16]

The biomechanical study by Curtis and colleagues[24] came to a similar conclusion as that of Politi and colleagues.[16] They found plate fixation to be the least rigid of all constructs, and the load needed for 1 mm and 2 mm of displacement to be the lowest with plate fixation compared with that of an interfragmentary screw and crossed K-wires. The investigators used a 5-hole or 6-hole tubular AO nonlocking plate with two 3.5-mm cortical screws into the metatarsal and two 3.5-mm cortical screws into the proximal phalanx.[24] The decreased biomechanical strength of the plate in comparison with the other forms of fixation was attributed to the nonideal positioning of the plate on the dorsal surface, rather than plantar surface, of the MTPJ.

Despite the increasing popularity of locking plates, there are no published studies of fusion rates of first MTPJ arthrodesis using this newer technique. In addition, no biomechanical studies are available comparing locking plates with nonlocking plates or other forms of fixation. This area needs further investigation.

Compression Screw with Plate

Recent research in both podiatric and orthopedic literature has looked at first MTPJ arthrodesis using a compression screw in conjunction with a nonlocking plate, as shown in **Fig. 3**, although the plate shown is a locking plate. Fusion rates are all comparable with other forms of fixation, leading to similar predictable clinical outcomes. Reported fusion rates range from 87.9% to 100%.[10–14] These studies reported low percentages of patients requiring hardware removal.[10–12]

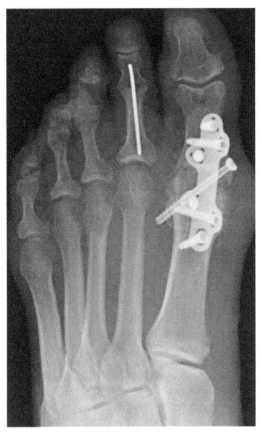

Fig. 3. Locking plate with interfragmentary compression screw. (*Courtesy of* Thomas A. Brosky, DPM, GA.)

Of the published studies of fusion rates, the plating systems used were nonlocking plates all made of titanium and 1 stainless steel system. In all studies, the compression screw was applied first,[10,11,13,14] except for 1 study in which the plate was applied before the compression screw.[12]

Sharma and colleagues[14] in 2008 compared use of a single compression screw with a compression screw with a one-quarter tubular plate. Thirty-four joints were fused, with no statistical difference in fusion rates. Also no difference in time to radiographic fusion was found. The investigators concluded that addition of a plate did not improve patient satisfaction or decrease complications, and therefore a plate is not needed as suggested by some biomechanical studies.

Only 2 biomechanical studies are available comparing a compression screw with a plate with other forms of fixation. Politi and colleagues[16] in 2003 found that use of a lag screw and plate was the most stable fixation construct compared with lag screw alone, crossed 0.062 K-wires, and a plate with no interfragmentary compression screw. The compression screw with plate was more than 2 times stronger than the lag screw alone, which was the next strongest construct ahead of the plate alone and crossed K-wires. The compression screw used was a 3.5-mm cortical lag screw and the plate was a 4-hole, vitallium, nonlocking plate secured with 3.5-mm cortical screws.

Buranosky and coleagues[34] compared the biomechanical strength of a plate with an interfragmentary screw with 2 crossed lag screws. They used a 6-hole Luhr nonlocking plate with 2.7-mm nonlocking screws. The central holes were eccentrically drilled to allow for compression. Once the plate was applied, the temporary K-wire crossing the joint was removed and replaced with a 2.7-mm cortical screw in lag fashion. In the other construct, 2 crossed 2.7-mm screws were used. The plate with interfragmentary screw construct was found to be a significantly stiffer form of fixation and failed at higher loads compared with a crossed-screw construct.[34]

More research is needed on this area. Locking plate technology seems to be absent from both biomechanical studies and clinical trials. Other variables, such as shape, material, and size (width and thickness), have not been addressed adequately to date.

Staple Fixation

The use of staples for first MTPJ arthrodesis is a recently introduced fixation option. Minimal research exists on this form of fixation. Rakesh and colleagues[15] in 2004 used 2 memory compression staples placed at right angles to each other. The staple used was composed of nitinol, an equiatomic nickel-titanium alloy. A fusion rate of 96.7% was achieved, which is comparable with other available forms of fixation.

Only 1 biomechanical study is available on staple fixation. Neufeld and colleagues[35] compared 3 different fixation methods: 2 crossed cannulated screws, a dorsal plate with an oblique 0.062 K-wire, and 2 compression staples with an oblique 0.062 K-wire. Staples provided the least stiffness and the least applied force to gap the fusion site compared with the other fixation methods in the study. The investigators recommended that, when using staples for first MTPJ arthrodesis, the patient be immobilized with a cast until union is achieved. In the previously mentioned study by Rakesh and colleagues,[15] postoperative cast immobilization was not used and only 1 nonunion occurred.[15]

Staples seem to be a reasonable fixation option considering the lack of studies available. More research is needed in this area. In addition to serving as the primary form of fixation, staples have the ability, like K-wires, to augment other forms of fixation, as shown in **Fig. 4**. **Fig. 5** shows an intraoperative image of a 2-staple box construct augmented with a longitudinally placed K-wire. Immediate postoperative and 1 year postoperative radiographs are shown in **Figs. 6** and **7**.

External Fixation

Little research has been done on the use of external fixation for first MTPJ arthrodesis. The biomechanical study by Sykes and Hughes[36] in 1986 compared screw fixation, external fixation, vertical wire suture, and horizontal wire suture as types of fixation for this procedure. They found that crossed-screw fixation techniques were able to maintain position of the fusion site the best when subjected to static loading. The external fixator was better at maintaining this position compared with the suture wire techniques.[36] The use of external fixation for first MTPJ arthrodesis is probably best when reserved for salvage cases in which bone graft is required and the patient has already had multiple surgical procedures on the first ray (**Fig. 8**).

Newer Fixation Options

At our institution a wide variety of fixation techniques for first MTPJ arthrodesis are used. Although traditional forms of fixation are still more frequently used, newer locking plate technology has been applied with good success. A 2-hole titanium locking miniplate has been a useful fixation device to augment and protect our primary form of fixation. **Fig. 9** shows a 3.8-mm headless cannulated compression screw

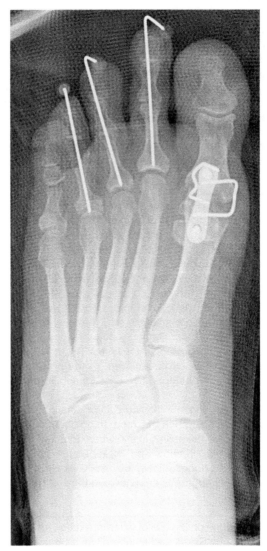

Fig. 4. Two-hole locking miniplate augmented with 2 staples. (*Courtesy of* Thomas A. Brosky, DPM, GA.)

augmented with the 2-hole locking miniplate. **Fig. 10** shows a crossed K-wire construct augmented with the same plate (**Fig. 4** shows staple fixation combined with this same plate). When greater stability is needed, such as for a noncompliant or obese patient, we use a larger locking plate, as shown in **Fig. 11**.

In 2010, McGlamry and Brosky[37] did a preliminary study on 10 patients having dorsally applied titanium locking plate and a box construct of 2 staples. Each construct was supplemented with either a K-wire or interfragmentary compression screw. Full weight bearing in the first week was allowed. All 10 patients went on to have solid fusions with no failure of fixation.[37]

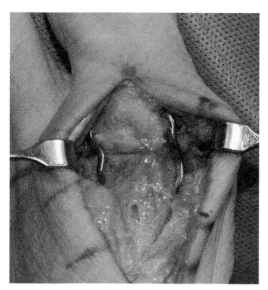

Fig. 5. Intraoperative image of 2-staple box construct augmented with a longitudinal K-wire.

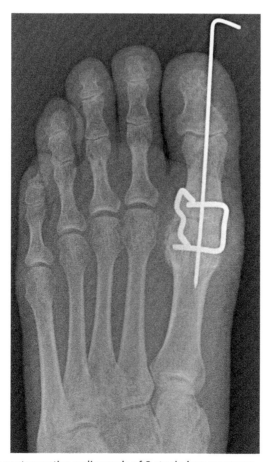

Fig. 6. Immediate postoperative radiograph of 2-staple box construct.

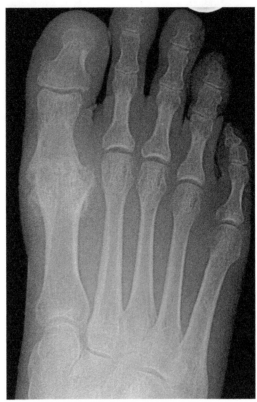

Fig. 7. One-year postoperative radiograph of 2-staple box construct after hardware removal.

DISCUSSION

This review examines evidence in the literature to establish whether one form of fixation should be recommended rather than another for first MTPJ arthrodesis. When reviewing the literature on published fusion rates, we found equally high rates for each type of fixation. Biomechanical studies tended to show increased strength and stability for more advanced forms of fixation such as screws alone and plates in conjunction with interfragmentary screws. Given the high fusion rates found clinically with all forms of fixation, it is difficult to make the recommendation that plate and screw constructs should be the accepted form of fixation. It is more appropriate to make recommendations on a smaller scale. For example, if a surgeon chooses to perform the procedure with K-wires, it may add to the stability of the fusion site if a K-wire is inserted longitudinally in addition to crossed K-wires rather than crossed K-wires alone. In addition, if a patient has an increased body mass index or will be weight bearing early in the postoperative course, then it may be appropriate to use more advanced forms of fixation such as screws and plates.

Although our analysis focused on fixation, we did encounter some additional findings, not related to fixation, of which surgeons should be aware. These findings are related to cost, hardware failure, and joint resection techniques.

Cost of surgical supplies is a growing concern in hospitals and surgical centers. There are a few studies in foot and ankle literature addressing the cost-

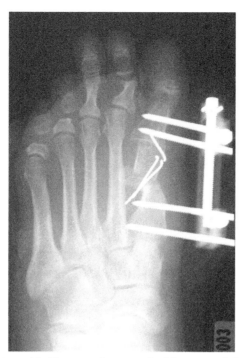

Fig. 8. External fixator with iliac crest bone graft. (*Courtesy of* George R. Vito, DPM, Las Vegas, NV.)

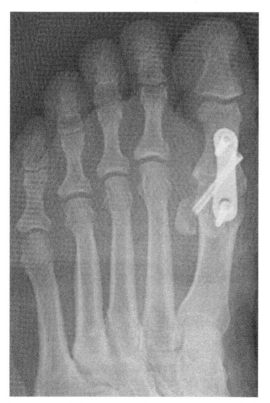

Fig. 9. Headless 3.8-mm cannulated compression screw augmented with 2-hole mini–locking plate. (*Courtesy of* Thomas A. Brosky, DPM, GA.)

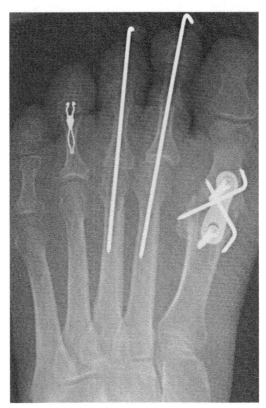

Fig. 10. Crossed 0.062 K-wires augmented with 2-hole mini–locking plate. (*Courtesy of* Thomas A. Brosky, DPM, GA.)

effectiveness of various fixation options when performing first MTPJ arthrodesis. Watson and Kelikian[38] found that AO screws had the lowest average cost and were the most cost-effective device for the procedure. Hyer and colleagues[8] compared cost of crossed-screw constructs with dorsal plating constructs. They found that 2 crossed screws were significantly less expensive than dorsal plating and, clinically, both systems gave similar acceptable results.

When choosing a type of fixation, evaluation of potential hardware failure is of concern. With the current fixation options available for first MTPJ arthrodesis, surgeons must choose between various sets of plates and screws. Most newer systems are made of titanium rather than stainless steel, which is a stronger material, although less biofriendly. Bennett and colleagues[32] performed 107 first MTPJ fusions using a titanium modular handset. They had a hardware failure rate of 13%, leading them to conclude that the titanium system that they used was not an ideal form of fixation for this procedure. More studies comparing stainless steel with titanium systems would be useful as surgical companies trend more toward titanium systems.

Although fixation is an important component of the procedure, joint preparation is of utmost importance. If the joint is not properly resected, then bony union may not occur even in the presence of the most stable fixation construct. There are different techniques for joint resection, such as conical reamers, planal (saw) resection, and curettage techniques. The goal of each technique is removal of all cartilage and subchondral plate such that cancellous bleeding bone is exposed. Some of the

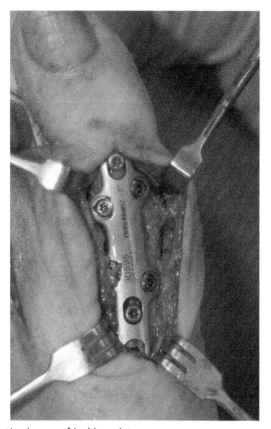

Fig. 11. Intraoperative image of locking plate.

biomechanical studies mentioned earlier compared the various joint resection techniques in addition to comparing the various fixation constructs. Politi and colleagues[16] studied joints fixated with a single lag screw and compared planal resected joints with conical reamed joints. Their results showed that the planal joint resection was significantly stronger than the reamed joint. Sykes and Hughes,[36] in a similar study, compared cancellous screw fixation in planal and conically resected joints and were able to make the same conclusion as Politi and colleagues[16]; planal joint resection is more stable for the studied fixation construct. The biomechanical study by Curtis and colleagues[24] also compared stability of planal resection versus reamer-prepared fusions as the studies by Politi and colleagues[16] and Sykes and Hughes[36] had done, and found that conical reaming of the joint was significantly more stable than planal resection of the joint. The investigators concluded that conical reaming creates a larger surface area for bone healing, which has an intrinsic stability that can be added to the stability that the fixation provides.[24] These studies show conflicting results regarding the proper way to prepare the joint for fusion, showing the need for more research in this area.

SUMMARY

High arthrodesis rates are found regardless of the type of fixation used. Biomechanical studies show a trend toward increased strength when more advanced forms of fixation, such as plates and screws, are used. The literature has yet to address the use of locking plate technology as a form of fixation for this procedure, which needs to be investigated.

REFERENCES

1. Mann RA, Coughlin MJ. Adult hallux valgus. In: Coughlin MJ, Mann RA, editors. Surgery of the foot and ankle. 7th edition. St Louis (MO): CV Mosby; 1999. p. 150–269.
2. Clutton HH. The treatment of hallux valgus. St Thomas Rep 1894;22:1.
3. McKeever D. Arthrodesis of the first metatarsophalangeal joint for hallux valgus, hallux rigidus, and metatarsus primus varus. J Bone Joint Surg Am 1952;34: 129–34.
4. Mann RA, Oates JC. Arthrodesis of the first metatarsophalangeal joint. Foot Ankle 1980;1:159–66.
5. Niskanen RO, Lehtimake MY, Hamalaiene MM, et al. Arthrodesis of the first metatarsophalangeal joint in rheumatoid arthritis. Acto Orthop Scand 1993;64:100–2.
6. Wassink S, Martin MD. Arthrodesis of the first metatarsophalangeal joint using a single screw: retrospective analysis of 109 feet. J Foot Ankle Surg 2009; 48(6):653–60.
7. Brodsky JW, Passmore RN, Pollo FE. Functional outcome of arthrodesis of the first metatarsophalangeal joint using parallel screw fixation. Foot Ankle Int 2005;26(2): 140–6.
8. Hyer CF, Glover JP, Berlet GC. Cost comparison of crossed screws versus dorsal plate construct for first metatarsophalangeal joint arthrodesis. J Foot Ankle Surg 2008;47(1):13–8.
9. Bennett MD, Sabetta J. First metatarsalphalangeal joint arthrodesis: evaluation of plate and screw fixation. Foot Ankle Int 2009;30(8):752–7.
10. Kumar S, Pradhan R, Rosenfeld PF. First metatarsophalangeal arthrodesis using a dorsal plate and a compression screw. Foot Ankle Int 2010;31(9):797–801.
11. Ellington JK, Carroll JP, Cohen BE, et al. Review of 107 hallux MTP joint arthrodesis using dome-shaped reamers and a stainless-steel dorsal plate. Foot Ankle Int 2010;31(5):385–90.
12. Goucher NR, Coughlin MJ. Hallux metatarsophalangeal joint arthrodesis using dome-shaped reamers and dorsal plate fixation: a prospective study. Foot Ankle Int 2006;27(11):869–76.
13. Flavin R, Stephen MM. Arthrodesis of the first metatarsophalangeal joint using a doral titanium contoured plate. Foot Ankle Int 2004;25(11):783–7.
14. Sharma H, Bhagat S, DeLeeuw J, et al. In vivo compression of screw versus plate and screw fixation for first metatarsophalangeal arthrodesis: does augmentation of internal compression screw fixation using a semi-tubular plate shorten time to clinical and radiologic fusion of the first metatarsophalangeal joint (MTPJ)? J Foot Ankle Surg 2008;47(1):2–7.
15. Rakesh CK, Theruvil B, Taylor GR. First metatarsophalangeal joint arthrodesis. A new technique of internal fixation by using memory compression staples. J Foot Ankle Surg 2004;43(5):312–7.
16. Politi J, Hayes J, Njus G, et al. First metatarsal-phalangeal joint arthrodesis: a biomechanical assessment of stability. Foot Ankle Int 2003;24(4):332–7.
17. Wyss UP, Mcbride I, Murphy L, et al. Joint reaction forces at the first MTP joint in a normal elderly population. J Biomech 1990;23:977–84.
18. Perren SM. Physical and biological aspects of fracture healing with special reverence to internal fixation. Clin Orthop 1975;138:175–95.

19. Sussman RE, Russo CT, Marquit H, et al. Arthrodesis of the first metatarsophalangeal joint. JAPMA 1986;76:631–5.
20. Coughlin MJ, Mann RA. Arthrodesis of the first metatarsophalangeal joint as a salvage for failed Keller procedure. J Bone Joint Surg Am 1987;69:68–74.
21. Fitzgerald JA. A review of long term results of arthrodesis o the first metatarsophalangeal joint. J Bone Joint Surg Br 1969;51:488–93.
22. Mann RA, Thompson FM. Arthrodesis of the first metatarsophalangeal joint for hallux valgus in rheumatoid arthritis. J Bone Joint Surg Am 1984;55:687–92.
23. Smith RW, Joainis TL, Maxwell PD. Great toe metatarsophalangeal joint arthrodesis: a user-friendly technique. Foot Ankle 1993;13:367.
24. Curtis MJ, Myerson M, Jinnah RH. Arthrodesis of the first metatarsophalangeal joint: a biomechanical study of internal fixation techniques. Foot Ankle 1993;14(7):395–9.
25. Rongstad KM, Miller GJ, Vander Griend RA, et al. A biomechanical comparison of four fixation methods of first metatarsophalangeal joint arthrodesis. Foot Ankle Int 1994;15(8):415–9.
26. Yu GV, Shook JE. Arthrodesis of the first metatarsophalangeal joint. JAPMA 1994;84(6):266–80.
27. Yu GV, Shook JE. Arthrodesis of the first metatarsophalangeal joint. In: Banks AS, Downey MS, Martin DE, et al, editors. McGlamry's comprehensive textbook of foot and ankle surgery. 3rd edition. Philadelphia: Lippincott Williams & Wilkins; 2001. p. 581–607.
28. Molloy S, Burkhart BG, Jasper LE. Biomechanical comparison of two fixation methods for first metatarsophalangeal joint arthrodesis. Foot Ankle Int 2003;24(2):169–71.
29. Hansen ST Jr. Arthrodesis techniques. In: Functional reconstruction of the foot and ankle. Philadelphia: Lippincott Williams & Wilkins; 2000. p. 283–356.
30. Ray RG. Methods of osseous fixation. In: Banks AS, Downey MS, Martin DE, et al, editors. McGlamry's comprehensive textbook of foot and ankle surgery. 3rd edition. Philadelphia: Lippincott Williams & Wilkins; 2001. p. 65–106.
31. Shaw JA. A biomechanical comparison of scaphoid screws. J Hand Surg Am 1987;12:347–53.
32. Bennett GL, Kay DB, Sabetta J. First metatarsal-phalangeal joint arthrodesis: evaluation of failure of hardware. Foot Ankle Int 2005;26(8):593–6.
33. Coughlin MJ, Abdo RV. Arthrodesis of the first metatarsophalangeal joint with vitallium plate fixation. Foot Ankle 1994;15(1):18–28.
34. Buranosky DJ, Taylor DT, Sage RA. First metatarsophalangeal joint arthrodesis: quantitative mechanical testing of six-hole dorsal plate versus crossed screw fixation in cadaveric specimens. J Foot Ankle Surg 2001;40(4):208–13.
35. Neufeld SK, Parks BG, Naseef GS, et al. Arthrodesis of the first metatarsophalangeal joint: a biomechanical study comparing memory compression staples, cannulated screws, and a dorsal plate. Foot Ankle Int 2002;23(2):97–101.
36. Sykes A, Hughes AW. A biomechanical study using cadaveric toes to test stability of fixation techniques employed in arthrodesis of the first metatarsophalangeal joint. Foot Ankle 1986;7(1):18–25.
37. McGlamry MC, Brosky TA. Analysis of early weight bearing following first metatarsophalangeal arthrodesis. In: Parker N, editor. Reconstructive surgery of the foot and leg: update 2010. Decatur (GA): Podiatry Institute; 2010. p. 175–7.
38. Watson AD, Kelikian AS. Cost-effectiveness comparison of three methods of internal fixation for arthrodesis of the first metatarsophalangeal joint. Foot Ankle Int 1998;19(5):304–10.

Primary Arthrodesis and Sural Artery Flap Coverage for Subtalar Joint Osteomyelitis in a Diabetic Patient

Crystal L. Ramanujam, DPM, Thomas Zgonis, DPM*

KEYWORDS

• Sural flap • Osteomyelitis • Diabetes mellitus • External fixation
• Ulcer

Tissue defects and osteomyelitis of the hindfoot and ankle often require creative strategies for complete resolution of infection and definitive wound closure. Limb salvage for diabetic patients faced with this clinical scenario is challenging because conservative and local treatments for infection usually fail. For osteomyelitis of the foot, staged reconstruction is recommended to effectively remove all grossly infected bone and soft tissue, followed by prolonged antibiotic therapy, and then final reconstructive procedures may be attempted.[1,2] These principles have long been followed for open fracture management in the lower extremity, and more recently have been extended to treatment of persistent bone and soft tissue infections resulting from other conditions, such as in the neuropathic lower extremity.[1,3–5] Realignment arthrodesis for chronic instability and associated deformities of the foot can provide the patient with a stable limb to withstand forces of ambulation. Wounds that are not amenable to traditional closure options can be addressed with more involved plastic surgical techniques, such as local, muscle, pedicle, or free flaps.[6] Before consideration for any reconstructive procedures, careful patient selection is required for an optimal outcome. This article describes an innovative case of limb salvage in the diabetic foot through treatment of subtalar joint osteomyelitis and associated wound using primary subtalar joint arthrodesis and coverage with the reverse sural artery neurofasciocutaneous flap.

Division of Podiatric Medicine and Surgery, Department of Orthopaedic Surgery, The University of Texas Health Science Center at San Antonio, 7703 Floyd Curl Drive–MSC 7776, San Antonio, TX 78229, USA
* Corresponding author.
E-mail address: zgonis@uthscsa.edu

Clin Podiatr Med Surg 28 (2011) 421–427
doi:10.1016/j.cpm.2011.02.003
0891-8422/11/$ – see front matter © 2011 Elsevier Inc. All rights reserved.

CASE REPORT

A 47-year-old man presented to the emergency department of our institution with redness, swelling, and pain to the right foot and ankle that had progressively worsened in the previous 2 weeks. He noticed a new draining wound to the side of the foot just below the ankle approximately 3 days earlier, which prompted him to seek medical attention. The condition was attributed to recent increase in activity with prolonged walking using inadequate shoegear despite a long history of foot ulcerations and previous amputations. His past medical history was significant for type 2 diabetes mellitus, peripheral neuropathy, hypertension, anemia, and Charcot neuroarthropathy of the right foot. The patient's surgical history included left foot partial first and second ray amputations as well as right foot partial fourth ray amputation and partial resection of the fifth metatarsal, with all procedures having been performed for treatment of osteomyelitis after chronic neuropathic ulcerations. He had no known drug allergies, denied alcohol use but admitted to a 30 pack-year history of smoking. He related a strong family history of diabetes mellitus, including multiple toe amputations in his father.

On initial presentation, the patient was a moderately obese man in no apparent distress and had stable vital signs. There was pitting edema to the right foot and ankle circumferentially but pedal pulses were palpable. A full-thickness wound was located at the lateral aspect of the foot that probed to bone and the subtalar joint with extensive periwound erythema and fluctuance. Purulence was expressible from the wound and there was significant pain on manipulation of the right foot and ankle. The patient had healed left partial first and second ray amputations, along with healed right partial fourth ray amputation with dorsal subluxation of the fifth digit at the metatarsophalangeal joint. The right foot also showed severe collapse at the midfoot and hindfoot secondary to Charcot neuroarthropathy. Plain film radiographs revealed soft tissue edema at the lateral aspect of the right foot and ankle with neuropathic degenerative changes about the midfoot and hindfoot; no osseous destruction was apparent. Magnetic resonance imaging of the right foot and ankle showed an abscess and hematoma formation along the lateral hindfoot and ankle. Laboratory analysis for complete blood cell count, serum chemistry, and urinalysis were within normal limits. The chest radiographs and electrocardiogram also showed no significant abnormality.

Because of evidence of abscess formation and suspicious osteomyelitis, urgent surgical decompression of the severe infection was required. Under general anesthesia, extensive debridement by sharp excision of all nonviable soft tissue was performed down to the level of the subtalar joint. Resection of grossly infected bone at the articular surfaces of the talus and calcaneus was performed. Deep soft tissue cultures of the wound were taken in addition to bone cultures and gross specimens from the talus and calcaneus were obtained, followed by copious irrigation of the site with 3000 mL of sterile normal saline through the pulse lavaging technique. The wound was packed open and the lower extremity was placed in a posterior splint to maintain stability of the right foot and ankle. The patient was admitted to the hospital in anticipation of further surgical procedures based on intraoperative culture and histopathology results. He was maintained on intravenous broad-spectrum antibiotics consisting of piperacillin-tazobactam and vancomycin. Final cultures of bone at the talus and calcaneus revealed growth of methicillin-resistant *Staphylococcus aureus* susceptible to vancomycin and tobramycin. Histopathologic examination of the talus and calcaneus specimens showed osteomyelitis. The patient was taken back to the operating room under local anesthesia for revisional debridement and insertion of tobramycin-loaded cement beads at the subtalar defect. The infectious disease service was consulted and recommended 6 weeks of vancomycin through a peripherally inserted central catheter for treatment of osteomyelitis. The patient was trained for non–weight bearing to the right foot with crutch assistance and was discharged to home 2 days later with the intravenous vancomycin and posterior splint to the right lower extremity. During his hospital stay, based on his history of diabetes and smoking, noninvasive vascular testing (including ankle-brachial index, toe-brachial index, pulse-volume recordings, and segmental pressures) was performed on both extremities to assess vascular status in preparation for any subsequent reconstruction. Results were significant only for increased ankle-brachial index caused by medial calcinosis of the vessels. Vascular surgery consultation was obtained to thoroughly evaluate the patient, and his status was deemed appropriate for further limb salvage. The patient was followed in the senior author's outpatient clinic every 2 weeks for the duration of the 6-week intravenous antibiotic therapy and had no complications. He was then readmitted to the hospital for surgical reconstruction. Initial surgery for the second hospital stay entailed removal of the antibiotic beads, sharp debridement of nonviable tissue to healthy bleeding, and deep soft tissue and bone cultures. The patient remained in the hospital on intravenous vancomycin, and final cultures revealed no growth of bacteria 4 days later.

The location of the wound at the lateral subtalar joint and the large defect from removal of bone at the initial surgeries lent themselves to a few options for definitive reconstruction; however, subtalar joint arthrodesis and coverage of the wound with a reverse sural artery flap was chosen. Vein mapping to the right lower extremity was performed before surgery to ensure patency of the lesser saphenous vein and mark its location at the posterior lower leg in preparation for dissection of the sural pedicle flap. General anesthesia was administered because of the extent of procedures planned. The patient was carefully placed in the prone position with appropriate padding to all osseous prominences of the body. A thigh tourniquet was secured to the right lower extremity and inflated to 350 mm Hg following exsanguination and povidone-iodine preparation of the entire limb. There was a 6-cm diameter full-thickness wound extending to the level of the bone at the subtalar joint, which was appropriately debrided to healthy tissue. The joint was prepared for fusion using a combination of curettes and osteotomes, removing all nonviable cartilage and bone. Multiple drill holes were made with a Steinmann pin to elicit good bleeding. Allogenic bone graft in the amount of 15 mL was placed within the subtalar joint. Stable fixation of the joint was achieved using multiple large Steinmann pins with fluoroscopic guidance to maintain appropriate alignment. Attention was then directed to harvesting of the sural artery pedicle flap. The shape of the defect at the wound was traced with a surgical marker onto sterile paper wrapping from the surgical gloves, cut out, and then retraced onto the proximal posterior leg. The medial sural nerve was identified followed by ligation of the median superficial sural artery and lesser saphenous vein each with 2 closely placed medium hemoclips. Isolation of the pedicle components was then performed after transection between the hemoclips. A Z-incision from the flap to the level of the soft tissue defect was performed using loupe magnification beginning proximal to distal, carefully protecting the neurovascular structures. The tourniquet was then released to assess flap viability and noted to be well perfused. The flap was turned down approximately 6 cm above the level of the ankle joint and inset into the recipient site at the subtalar joint defect. Care was taken not to kink the pedicle. The flap was secured to the wound using 3-0 nylon and the donor site was primarily closed using 3-0 nylon. A meshed split-thickness skin graft obtained from the lateral aspect of the right leg was then used to cover the neurovascular pedicle. The patient was then repositioned from prone to supine on the operating table and the limb was reprepped and draped. A modified Ilizarov circular external fixator system was then applied to the right foot and ankle for off-loading and stabilization of the right lower extremity. The leg was carefully dressed to avoid covering the pedicle flap to allow for postoperative inspection (**Fig. 1**).

The patient was kept in the hospital for bedrest during the first 48 hours, during which deep vein thrombosis prophylaxis was enforced through a pneumatic compression device to the contralateral limb and daily administration of low–molecular-weight heparin directed by the medical team. The flap was inspected every 2 hours for the first 24 hours, and then every 4 to 6 hours for the next 48 hours, for evidence of ischemia or venous congestion. The patient was slowly progressed through physical therapy for non–weight bearing to the right lower extremity using assistive devices during the next 4 days before discharge from the hospital. The patient was released with a 2-week oral course of the culture-specific antibiotic doxycycline. The senior author followed the patient in the outpatient setting every 2 weeks for 8 weeks to check viability of the flap and evaluate the arthrodesis site through serial radiographs. The patient's postoperative course was uneventful, and the modified Ilizarov external fixator and Steinmann pins were removed at 9 weeks after the staged reconstruction. The patient's affected limb was placed into a well-padded short leg cast and he maintained non–weight bearing status to the right foot for 6 additional weeks. The flap had complete incorporation at the recipient site and complete union of the subtalar arthrodesis was noted, therefore he was progressed to assisted weight bearing in a removable surgical boot for 6 weeks. He was then placed into custom-molded extra-depth shoes with accommodative inlays. At the last follow-up visit 28 weeks after reconstruction, the patient was able to successfully ambulate on the foot with maintenance of durable closure to all surgical sites.

DISCUSSION

Large tissue defects and bone loss following treatment of infectious conditions in the foot often leave surgeons with few options for resolution other than amputation. The functional demands and expectations of the patient should be reasonably explored to ensure that reconstruction is more beneficial than amputation.[7] Appropriate patient selection is further based on a thorough review of the patient's medical history, taking into account all comorbid conditions such as diabetes mellitus, renal impairment, and cardiovascular disease. Patients should be counseled on modifiable risk factors including smoking and glycemic control. A complete review of the patient's history of lower extremity surgeries, including each postoperative course, is critical to identify potential complications that may be encountered with further reconstructive attempts. For example, prior antibiotic use may give clues to drug resistance in the infected joint and aid in selection of perioperative antibiotics.[1] Formal vascular evaluation of the lower extremities is imperative to determine whether limb salvage is possible and whether revascularization procedures may be necessary to facilitate successful reconstruction. Appropriate imaging, such as radiographs, magnetic resonance, computed tomography, or specific bone scans, of the lower extremity based on the clinical presentation is vital for preoperative planning.[8] A multidisciplinary approach is ideal for perioperative management, including internists, infectious disease specialists, vascular surgeons, plastic surgeons, nursing staff, wound care specialists, physical therapists, and nutritionists.[2]

Extensive irrigation and debridement of devitalized bone and soft tissue is performed to initially address the infection. If positive bone cultures result, prolonged parenteral antibiotics tailored to the sensitivities identified may be required for 6 to

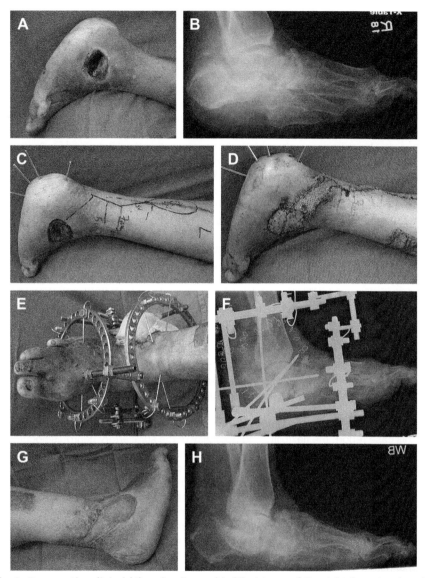

Fig. 1. Preoperative clinical (*A*) and radiographic (*B*) pictures of the right foot showing the large defect of the subtalar joint after removal of the antibiotic cemented beads and aggressive debridement. Intraoperative picture (*C*) showing the stabilization of the subtalar joint with large Steinmann pins as well as the drawing on the posterior aspect of the leg for harvesting the pedicle flap. Intraoperative picture (*D*) showing the insetting of the reverse flow sural neurofasciocutaneous flap into the recipient area of the prepared subtalar joint arthrodesis. The donor site on this case was primarily closed and a split-thickness skin graft was harvested from the lateral aspect of the lower leg to cover the pedicle area and to avoid any skin tension over the neurovascular bundle (*D*). Postoperative clinical (*E*) and radiographic (*F*) pictures showing the modified Ilizarov circular external fixator for stabilization and off-loading of the pedicle flap. Long-term clinical (*G*) and radiographic (*H*) pictures at 28-week follow-up.

8 weeks for suppression of osteomyelitis.[4,5] During this time, local delivery of antibiotics can be facilitated with the use of antibiotic-loaded cement beads. A heat-stable antibiotic must be chosen with microbial coverage specific to the patient's wound cultures and according to recommendations from the infectious disease specialist.[9–11] In cases of joint sepsis and contiguous osteomyelitis, particularly involving the subtalar joint, appropriate resection of nonviable bone can result in severe instability to the foot and ankle. Fusion of the subtalar joint using appropriate fixation techniques can provide a stable, plantigrade foot and also facilitates adequate muscle and tendon function at the ankle. Stabilization of the bone segments also eliminates abnormal soft tissue motion and irritation.[1,12] Choice of fixation used in the arthrodesis is important. In this case report, because of the patient's history of multiple infections, soft tissue compromise, and decreased bone density, external fixation and Steinmann pins were used as opposed to internal fixation. Furthermore, joint compression techniques using external fixation can assist with arthrodesis, and the construct allows for regular monitoring of soft tissue reconstruction.[13]

Without durable closure of the adjacent soft tissue envelope, underlying osseous procedures are subject to complications, particularly recurring infection. Because all devitalized soft tissue must be removed to initially treat the infection, primary closure is not always possible; likewise, skin grafts and local flaps may also be inadequate for complete coverage of the defect. Pedicle or muscle flaps and free tissue transfer are viable options for large wounds at the lower extremity.[6] For the hindfoot and ankle in particular, muscle flaps have limited use because of location; in addition, free tissue transfer is more technically difficult to perform, requires longer operating times, and is associated with increased morbidity.[14] The reverse flow sural artery neurofasciocutaneous flap, originally described by Masquelet and colleagues,[15] has been reported to be useful for wound coverage in the diabetic foot.[2,14–16] This pedicle flap is distally based using the median superficial sural artery and nerve and has been reliably applied for wounds located at the plantar or posterior aspect of the calcaneus.[6,17] For this case report, the flexibility and durability of the sural artery neurofasciocutaneous flap allowed for optimal coverage of the patient's defect. Familiarity of anatomy and angiology, in addition to meticulous surgical technique, is crucial to the successful use of the sural artery neurofasciocutaneous flap. The authors use preoperative vascular imaging with vein mapping to pinpoint the exact location of the pedicle and determine the diameter of the lesser saphenous vein.[2] Known complications of the this pedicle flap are wound dehiscence, flap necrosis, venous congestion, and late skin breakdown. A vein diameter of greater than 2 mm is preferred to ensure patency and prevent venous congestion.[17] Medicinal leeches have been reported to be effective in the treatment of venous congestion.[18] In addition, the use of external fixation as seen in this case report to off-load the flap decreases the likelihood of complications and flap failure.[16,19]

SUMMARY

Diabetic limb salvage for chronic wounds and osteomyelitis of the diabetic foot requires a systematic approach focused on thorough preoperative evaluation, precise intraoperative technique, and diligent postoperative care. Following eradication of infection, combined subtalar joint fusion and coverage with the sural artery neurofasciocutaneous flap can achieve a functional, plantigrade foot with a durable soft tissue envelope that can be accommodated with conventional shoe gear.

REFERENCES

1. Baumhauer JF, Lu AP, DiGiovanni BF. Arthodesis of the infected ankle and subtalar joint. Foot Ankle Clin 2002;7:175–90.
2. Zgonis T, Stapleton JJ, Rodriguez RH, et al. Plastic surgery reconstruction of the diabetic foot. AORN J 2008;87:951–66.
3. Kitaoka HB, Patzer GL. Arthrodesis for the treatment of arthrosis of the ankle and osteonecrosis of the talus. J Bone Joint Surg Am 1998;80:370–9.
4. Cierny G, Cook WG, Mader JT. Ankle arthrodesis in the presence of ongoing sepsis. Indications, methods and results. Orthop Clin North Am 1989;20:709–21.
5. Richter D, Hahn MP, Laun RA, et al. Arthrodesis of the infected ankle and subtalar joint: technique, indications, and results of 45 consecutive cases. J Trauma 1999; 47:1072–8.
6. Rohmiller MT, Callahan BS. The reverse sural neurocutaneous flap for hindfoot and ankle coverage: experience and review of the literature. Orthopedics 2005; 28(12):1449–53.
7. Malizos KN, Gougoulias NE, Dailiana ZH, et al. Ankle and foot osteomyelitis: treatment protocol and clinical results. Injury 2010;41:285–93.
8. Dinh T, Snyder G, Veves A. Review papers: current techniques to detect foot infection in the diabetic patient. Int J Low Extrem Wounds 2010;9:24–30.
9. Chen NT, Hong HZ, Hooper DC, et al. The effect of systemic antibiotic and antibiotic impregnated polymethylmethacrylate beads on the bacterial clearance in wounds containing contaminated dead bone. Plast Reconstr Surg 1993;9: 1305–11.
10. Donati D, Biscaglia R. The use of antibiotic impregnated cement in infected reconstructions after resection for bone tumours. J Bone Joint Surg Br 1998;80: 1045–50.
11. Popham GJ, Mangino P, Seligson D, et al. Antibiotic impregnated beads: part II: factors in antibiotic selection. Orthop Rev 1991;20:331–7.
12. Zalavras CG, Patzakis MJ, Thordarson DB, et al. Infected fractures of the distal tibial metaphysis and plafond. Clin Orthop Relat Res 2004;427:57–62.
13. Belczyk R, Ramanujam CL, Capobianco CM, et al. Combined midfoot arthrodesis, muscle flap coverage, and circular external fixation for the chronic ulcerated Charcot deformity. Foot Ankle Spec 2010;3:40–4.
14. Kneser U, Bach AD, Polykandriotis E, et al. Delayed reverse sural flap for staged reconstruction of the foot and lower leg. Plast Reconstr Surg 2005;116:1910–7.
15. Masquelet AC, Romana MC, Wolf G. Skin island flaps supplied by the vascular axis of the sensitive superficial nerves: anatomic study and clinical experience in the leg. Plast Reconstr Surg 1992;89:1115–21.
16. Baumeister SP, Spierer R, Erdmann D, et al. Realistic complication analysis of 70 sural artery flaps in a multimorbid patient group. Plast Reconstr Surg 2003;112: 129–40.
17. Zgonis T, Stapleton JJ, Papakostas I. Local and distant pedicle flaps for soft tissue reconstruction of the diabetic foot: a stepwise approach with the use of external fixation. In: Zgonis T, editor. Surgical reconstruction of the diabetic foot and ankle. Philadelphia: Lippincott Williams & Wilkins; 2009. p. 178–92.
18. Mamelak AJ, Jackson A, Nizamani R, et al. Leech therapy in cutaneous surgery and disease. J Drugs Dermatol 2010;9:252–7.
19. Noack N, Hartmann B, Kuntscher MV. Measures to prevent complications of distally based neurovascular sural flaps. Ann Plast Surg 2006;57:37–40.

Index

Note: Page numbers of article titles are in **boldface** type.

Clin Podiatr Med Surg 28 (2011) 429–439
doi:10.1016/S0891-8422(11)00035-8
0891-8422/11/$ – see front matter © 2011 Elsevier Inc. All rights reserved.

podiatric.theclinics.com

Moving?

Make sure your subscription moves with you!

To notify us of your new address, find your **Clinics Account Number** (located on your mailing label above your name), and contact customer service at:

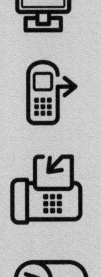

Email: journalscustomerservice-usa@elsevier.com

800-654-2452 (subscribers in the U.S. & Canada)
314-447-8871 (subscribers outside of the U.S. & Canada)

Fax number: 314-447-8029

Elsevier Health Sciences Division
Subscription Customer Service
3251 Riverport Lane
Maryland Heights, MO 63043

*To ensure uninterrupted delivery of your subscription, please notify us at least 4 weeks in advance of move.

Printed and bound by CPI Group (UK) Ltd, Croydon, CR0 4YY

03/10/2024

01040446-0005